Bernie Nolan

Now and Forever

Hodder & Stoughton Ltd
338 Euston Road
London NW1 3BH

www.hodder.co.uk

HODDER

First published in Great Britain in 2013 by Hodder & Stoughton
An Hachette UK company

First published in paperback in 2013

1

A CIP catalogue record for this title is available from the British Library

Paperback ISBN 978 1 444 77680 5
Ebook ISBN 978 1 444 77681 2

Typeset in Sabon LT Std by Palimpsest Book Production Limited
Falkirk, Stirlingshire

Printed and bound by CPI Group (UK) Ltd, Croydon, CR0 4YY

Hodder & Stoughton policy is to use papers that are natural, renewable
and recyclable products and made from wood grown in sustainable
forests. The logging and manufacturing processes are expected to conform
to the environmental regulations of the country of origin.

For my darling Steve and Erin. I dedicate this book to you – my two heroes. I love you both more than life itself xxxxx

CONTENTS

....

PROLOGUE

....

'We've got a long, hard fight ahead of us, Bernie, but we can do it,' said my consultant Mark Kissin, as I sobbed in his arms. It was April 2012 and I was sitting in his office at the Royal Surrey County Hospital. I'd just found out that the breast cancer I'd fought so hard to beat had come back – and that it had spread to my lungs, liver, bones and brain. And that there was no cure. It was devastating and I was scared. Nothing can prepare you for that kind of news. Suddenly, everything seems unfamiliar and you're staring down the barrel of a gun at a future that's horribly certain, but you have no idea what the journey there will hold for you.

They would treat me with drugs to try to contain the cancer and keep me alive for as long as possible, but that was all they could do. It was a very bleak prognosis. Still, I'd been told my condition was 'treatable' – that was the word my consultant used, and to my mind it was a million times better than saying nothing could be done for me. Believe it or not, I consider myself a lucky person because I was born an optimist. My glass has always been half full and I'm passionate about life. So I made the decision right from the start that I'd rather live with hope than be told I had six months or a year or five years to live. How could I carry on like that, watching the days and months tick by, waiting to die? 'You might as well get it over with now, Doc!' would have been my reply.

My positivity has been crucial in helping me to live with cancer and win many little battles along the way. I would be lying if I said I never had dark moments when I felt scared and desperate and sad, but I never once thought of myself as 'dying of cancer' – my attitude has always been that I'm living with it.

I also believe the experiences that shaped my childhood and teenage years armed me with many of the qualities I needed to take on this disease: a fighting spirit, determination, a rebellious streak and a bloody good sense of humour. Being born into a family of eight kids – with five very competitive sisters – meant I always had to shout louder than the rest to get myself heard. And being part of a sweet and innocent girl band with an overly strict father at the helm also gave me plenty to rebel against! Not bad preparation for summoning up the sheer bloody-mindedness you need when you're trying to beat the odds of a pretty grim cancer diagnosis and get your doctors to listen to you.

I've never been the kind of girl to give up on things easily, which probably comes from being in showbiz since the age of two. I have very few childhood memories that don't involve a costume change! One thing the showbiz school of hard knocks taught me was to get up, dust myself down and soldier on. And since being diagnosed with cancer three years ago, that's exactly what I've been doing.

But what motivates me more than anything to keep fighting is my family – my wonderful husband Steve and our gorgeous daughter Erin. I've taken so much strength from them. Steve has always been there for me – over the years he's made many sacrifices for my career and he's been my rock throughout this illness.

And I would never have managed to fight the way I have without Erin's amazing maturity, and I'm more determined than ever to be here for her. I desperately want to see her grow into the beautiful woman I know she will be. I have to see it! People have called me brave, but I'm more determined than brave. I'm just terrified I might die and miss something important in Erin's life. For that reason alone, I will never stop fighting.

It never entered my head that I was writing a memoir because I was going to die – quite the opposite. I want this book to be a celebration of my life, which has been full, happy, exciting and filled with wonderful people and experiences. Cancer is a relatively new thing for me and, yes, it has changed me – how could it not? But I don't want to be thought of as 'Cancer Girl'. I don't want the disease to define me.

Cancer has become part of my journey, but it's not the whole story. There's so much more to me than that. I'm a wife, mother, daughter, singer, actress, sister, friend and auntie – those are the roles I want to define me.

And I love this life of mine far too much to let it go without a fight, so bring it on.

1
ACROSS THE IRISH SEA TO BLACKPOOL

....

It's close to midnight on a Thursday in mid-December 1966 and I'm sitting on the dusty floor of a freezing cold dressingroom, my eyes still stinging from the smoky concert room we've just performed in. We've had a great night; the audience loved our show and stood up to cheer and applaud us. But now we're all exhausted – Mum and my brothers and sisters and I – and we're waiting patiently for Dad to drive us home to Blackpool. He's holding court at the bar with the club chairman and committee members, downing his umpteenth brandy of the night. I'm only six years old and I have to get up for school the next morning.

It was an all too familiar scenario during my childhood. As part of The Singing Nolans, I performed almost every night at working men's clubs and talent shows across the North of England. We were always hanging around after the show, waiting for my dad to finish his drink so we could go home to bed. There were no motorways back then and sometimes we'd travel as far afield as North Wales, which meant driving back in the dark along bumpy winding roads in a rickety old van. My dad never thought twice about getting behind the wheel of his van drunk, with eight kids crammed into the back. I often wondered why my mum let him get away with it, but as I got older I realised she was scared of confronting him. Occasionally, she'd challenge him about keeping us up late and we'd all plead with her: 'Mum, please just leave it!'

'I won't leave it!' she'd say defiantly, then Dad would lean across to the passenger seat and give her a backhander, and she'd be in floods of tears. She loved my dad a great deal, but there was no question he was the boss.

When we eventually did get home to our little four-bedroom terraced house in Waterloo Road, Blackpool, we'd all scurry upstairs, desperate to fall into bed. I usually slept in my tights in winter because it was so cold in the bedroom – we had no central heating in those days.

Often my mum wouldn't go to bed at all – she had to be up at 6 a.m. anyway to get us ready for school. So she'd build a fire for the morning and put all our school shirts on a clothes horse in front of it to warm them up, then she'd make a huge pan of porridge for breakfast before getting seven of us up for school.

Sometimes after we'd gone to bed, we could hear our parents shouting at each other downstairs and often we'd hear a crack, and it was obvious that Dad had slapped my mum. It was horrible, lying in bed listening to the row with the blankets pulled up tightly under my chin, wishing it would stop.

Although it wasn't the most glamorous start in show business, it really wasn't all bad – far from it. Even as a tiny child, I loved being on stage. I got so much joy from singing and performing, and that has stayed with me all my life. It just felt like the most natural thing in the world.

My parents Tommy and Maureen were thirty-four when I came into the world, on 17 October 1960. They named me Bernadette Therese Nolan. They'd already had six children – Tommy, my eldest brother was eleven, then came Anne, ten, Denise, eight, Maureen, six, Brian, five, and Linda, who was just twenty months. In Ireland back then we were actually considered a small family – our next-door neighbours had sixteen kids!

I was just 6lbs at birth, and my brothers and sisters were all crazy about me when Mum brought me home because I looked like a little doll. My sister Denise took it upon herself to be a kind of surrogate mum and she did everything for me, from changing my nappy to taking me out for walks. I've been told that sometimes if Mum and Denise held their arms out to me, I'd run to Denise first. I suppose we were typical of families where there's a big age gap between kids – the older ones have to muck in to help. As we grew up, we naturally fell into three groups: the Boys, the Big Girls (Anne, Denise and Maureen) and the Kids (Linda and I, and Coleen when she came along in 1965).

I don't have many memories of our house in Maryville Road, Dublin, because we moved to Blackpool when I was just two, but my best friend was also called Bernie and we used to play out in the street together. I vividly remember standing in front of a manhole cover on our street with Bernie one day, trying to work out how we could remove it so we could jump down and see what was there. Early signs of an inquisitive mind and a spirit of adventure!

I also remember my mum tying dusters around our feet and putting polish on them, then we'd all skip around the house polishing the wooden floors for her. We didn't have a lot of money – our house was a modest three-up, two-down semi on a council estate – but my mum kept it immaculate. She was incredibly house-proud and was always out polishing the front step.

She kept herself pristine, too. She had a lovely figure and beautiful Irish colouring – jet-black hair and green eyes. She seemed unbelievably glamorous and reminded me of Elizabeth Taylor.

I adored her. She was a wonderful woman and an amazing mum – very affectionate and always there for a cuddle. She was also an incredibly talented singer and at seventeen won a place to train as a soprano at the Dublin College of Music, but she never took it up. Instead, she started performing in clubs around the city, which is how she met my dad. He was known as Dublin's Sinatra and he actually looked a lot like him, too – short and slight with dark hair. And he had a fantastic voice. He ended up singing with his own dance band at a Dublin ballroom and became something of a heart-throb – the girls in the audience used to throw their underwear at him and scream, 'We love you, Tommy!'

My mum and dad hadn't been seeing each other long when she fell pregnant with my brother Tommy. But having a child outside marriage was unthinkable for a Catholic girl in Dublin in the late forties, so they hatched a plan to go to London and have the baby there. Mum went ahead and found a B&B to stay in and Dad said he'd meet her there in a few days' time, but he never showed up. It must have been terrifying and heartbreaking for my mum to realise that he'd abandoned her. In the end, the woman who ran the B&B got in touch with Mum's parents and her dad went to London to bring her home, saying they'd help her to bring up the baby.

Once my mum was back in Ireland, though, my dad asked her to marry him. I'm not sure if he did it because he thought it was the decent thing to do or if he was told, 'You're marrying her!' but I don't believe it's what he really wanted. And I think he rebelled against his fate for years afterwards.

They got married at a register office in 1948, but there are no photographs of the day. None of us even knew the story of Mum running away until we'd grown up and left home.

My parents had a shared passion for singing, though, and they started performing duets around the Dublin clubs. They were known as Tommy and Maureen, the Sweethearts of Song. But the difference in their personalities was obvious from the beginning. My dad liked to hang out in bars and he loved to drink and smoke – I always remember him spitting out little bits of tobacco from un-tipped cigarettes. My mum liked to socialise too, but she preferred to have people over to our house for dinner or a party. I suppose my dad was a bit of a Jack the Lad, and later on he had affairs that broke my mum's heart. Even as a kid I remember feeling sorry for Mum because she never got back the love she deserved and longed for, not until the very end when my dad was ill and he realised how much he loved her. I don't ever remember them kissing or holding hands. There was a real lack of affection between them, which seemed very sad.

In 1962 my parents decided to move us all to Blackpool. A friend of my dad's, who we called Uncle Fred, convinced him that there were lots of opportunities for singers. In those days, Blackpool was the centre of showbiz – it had a thriving entertainment industry – so we boarded the ferry and crossed the Irish Sea to a new life in England. Mum bought Linda and me new yellow dresses and coats with matching straw boaters for the trip, which was a real novelty as our clothes were usually hand-me-downs from our older sisters. I was only two years old and Linda was three, so we must have looked very cute.

At first, Uncle Fred put us up in his small terraced house in Ascot Road, which must have been a shock to his system. He was a single man who was used to living on his own and suddenly he was inundated with kids!

Anne hadn't come with us. She'd been diagnosed with a heart condition, so my parents made the decision to leave her in Ireland in a convalescent home. When I was older, I thought it was a strange decision for them to leave their twelve-year-old daughter behind while they relocated to another country, but I suppose they felt it was better for her to get well before making the trip. However, when she joined us in Blackpool six months later, the doctors said there was nothing seriously wrong with her and that she just had a very slight heart murmur.

We ended up staying with Uncle Fred for a couple of years and we loved our time there. He was a lovely man – very kind and patient, which was just as well!

Dad had several jobs on the go to earn enough money to keep us all – he worked as a bookkeeper in an accountant's office and laboured on a farm, too. Then at night he'd put on his tux and go out singing with Mum around the clubs in Blackpool. I used to love watching Mum apply her make-up at the dressingtable before going out to sing – putting kohl liner around her eyes and setting her beehive with lacquer from a little squeezy bottle. She always wore a beautiful long evening dress and Tweed perfume, and I used to breathe in the musky fragrance when she bent down to kiss me goodnight.

And it wasn't long before I performed to a proper audience for the first time. I was still only two when I made my debut at the Peter Webster show at the end of the pier. It was a talent competition and I sang 'Show Me the Way to Go Home' – and won! The prize was a gold watch and I sold it to my mum for three pence. When I decided I wanted it back, she said, 'Oh no, Bernie, we had a deal.' She wasn't stupid!

I'm amazed my first performance was such a success because I was a painfully shy child, which my friends now find hard to believe. But I used to hide behind my mum whenever we had guests at the house and she'd have to coax me to come out and say hello. My sisters tell me I was very sweet at that age – a tiny little thing with fair hair (which my dad cut himself using a bowl), bright blue eyes and pale skin.

Just before Coleen was born in March 1965, we moved out of Uncle Fred's into our own house on Waterloo Road. It was a four-up, two-down in a terrace, and it had to accommodate all ten of us. I was very excited that Mum was going to have another baby, but when Coleen was born I actually felt a bit put out. When we went singing I used to be the one to sit on Mum's knee in the car, but when Coleen came along she got pride of place on her knee and I was relegated to sitting beside her! Coleen was gorgeous though, and I used to kiss her and pinch her cheeks all the time, which drove her nuts. 'No, Bernie!' she'd squeal.

We all had to share bedrooms – I didn't have my own room until I was twenty-five! I was in with Linda and Coleen, the three big girls shared a room and so did my brothers, and my dad had his own room, which meant Mum had to sleep on the couch downstairs. I loved my dad, but he was a male chauvinist and my mum just put up with it. He used to dismiss her opinions and tell her to shut up all the time, and at dinner time she had to serve my dad and my brothers first.

Mum did everything for us. She'd cook three or four different meals a night and did all the washing-up afterwards. She was forever cleaning the house and doing our laundry. I feel ashamed now that none of us helped more, but she loved being a mum and was devoted to us. Naturally, she'd feel stressed and overwhelmed sometimes, and she'd scream and shout at us. She was an Irish woman after all and we do a lot of shouting, but our bark is worse than our bite!

* * *

At the time, I felt sad that she never had a moment to sit down and look at my homework with me or just talk to me. When I got older I thanked God I had elder sisters to tell me about periods and boys because my mum never had a spare minute to have those conversations. Her days were taken up with running the house and at night she was out performing with us – The Singing Nolans. During our show, which used to last about two hours, she'd sing a bit of opera and Dad did a few Sinatra songs. We all sang harmonies together on songs from shows like *Mary Poppins* and *The Sound of Music*. Tommy played the drums and the rest of us sang solos. My big number was the Flanagan and Allen song 'Strolling' and I wore a straw hat and a little blazer.

We began to get a name for ourselves, not just in the pubs and theatres across the North-West, but as far afield as Scotland and Wales – we used to perform there during the school holidays – and in London, too. When I was about six we started performing with the Showmen's Guild at the Grosvenor House hotel in London. The audience was full of rich people, all dressed up in their finery. When I sang 'Strolling' in my little blazer and straw boater, they all threw money at me! I got about £100 the first time, which was a fortune in those days. We did other gigs at posh hotels in London and we'd pull up in our van and all pile out like the Clampetts from *The Beverly Hillbillies*, carrying plastic bags stuffed with our belongings. The doorman would often come up to my dad and say, 'Can I help you?' really snootily, and we'd say, 'Yeah we're working, actually! We're The Singing Nolans.' Then he'd usher us in through a side entrance to keep us out of the way. I was too young to get the snobbery – I just found it funny. And I guess we must have looked a right sight pulling up outside such smart venues in this bloody big van!

There were plenty more cringeworthy episodes from our travels. We used to perform at a Labour club in Wigan and a friend called Nellie, who always came to cheer us on, offered my dad her old dining table. So my dad strapped this huge table to the roof of his old estate car and proceeded to drive down the motorway, where it promptly fell off. It must have looked hilarious, but I felt completely traumatised at the time because my dad went back to pick it up and I was convinced he was going to get run over.

We started performing at the Brunswick Club in Blackpool around the time that laws came in preventing younger children working after 9 p.m., so Linda and I couldn't stay for the whole show. At first we were absolutely disgusted, but after a while we began to like it because friends of my parents used to pick us up and take us home, and we'd get fish and chips on the way, and get to bed early so we were fresh for school the next day.

I loved being on stage, but I hated all the travelling to and from gigs, and all the hanging around after the show. And I hated the feeling of going to school dog-tired the next morning. Now I have my own child, I can't quite imagine where my parents' heads were at! I think they felt that at least we were all together as a family, but they must have known deep down that it was wrong to keep us up so late and send us to school exhausted.

Mum and Dad weren't bad parents though – it didn't feel like that at all to me. On the whole, I had a happy childhood and I was a very happy kid because I got to sing. We were never around to go to youth clubs and do things with our mates, which I resented a bit. I'd have a moan sometimes, but I got over it. It might not have been a normal childhood, but it was my childhood and I guess it made me the person I am today.

And Dad did let me off singing if there was something I really wanted to do. I was very sporty at school and I remember coming home one day and asking if I could go to a netball rally instead of performing and he let me. I think he was a bit stricter with the older girls, but I figured I was owed some time off – they hadn't been singing since the age of two like I had!

One of the things my parents did for us was to make sure we had a proper summer holiday every year. Those were the times when we could just be normal kids and have fun. They paid money into a holiday scheme at the Brunswick Club, then at the end of the season we'd go to somewhere like Benidorm. I was seven or eight when we first went to Spain and it was a really big deal because we hadn't been abroad before. We had lots of fun on those holidays. I had my first crush in Benidorm! Linda and I were in love with the sons of one of the club's committee members. And every year the kids would have a fancy-dress party and I always dressed as someone before and after marriage – one side of me was all glam and smart, and on the other side I wore half an apron and a slipper, and looked really dishevelled. It was hilarious! Those were good times.

I have wonderful memories of the years we spent at Waterloo Road, but it held some bad memories too. I hated the way my dad treated my mum, and I especially hated the fact that he could be violent, too, and hit her many times. Seeing that growing up definitely affected my relationships later in life and I could never have remained in a relationship where I wasn't considered an equal by my partner.

Dad was a Jekyll and Hyde character. When he was out drinking, everyone loved him – he was the life and soul. Everyone wanted to be in Tommy's gang or on Tommy's table. But if he got home in a bad mood with a drink inside him, there was hell to pay. It was horrible listening to him shout at my mum. Times like that, I felt like I didn't know him. He seemed like a different person to the dad I loved.

Mum never ended up in hospital or had broken bones – thank God – but I remember her having a fat lip a few times and I'd see bruises on her arms from where he'd punched her. It was disgusting and really hard to make sense of as a kid. I have a memory of him kicking her in the leg once after a show and seeing the gash forming and blood pouring out of it. It was a horrific thing for a small child to see. That time it started because he'd been drinking heavily and Mum was saying that he shouldn't be driving home drunk.

My eldest brother Tommy used to try to stick up for Mum and step in when they were fighting. One time Anne was having a row with my dad over something petty – they were sitting in armchairs in our living-room at Waterloo Road – and she wouldn't back down. He gave

her a backhander across the face and her lip burst open
and started bleeding.

We were all saying, 'Anne, just say you're sorry! Just
say you didn't mean it!' because we were frightened of
things escalating.

'No, I won't! I'm not wrong, he's wrong!' she screamed.
Whack! He hit her again.

'I'm not saying I'm sorry!' *Whack!* She got another
backhander. She ended up with a huge fat lip and when
my brother came home later that day she tried to hide
it from him, but no amount of make-up could disguise it.

'What the hell's happened?' asked Tommy when he
caught sight of Anne's lip. 'Did Dad do that to you?
The bastard! I'm going to kill him!'

'Just leave it, Tommy,' pleaded Anne. 'It just makes it
worse.'

When Dad came home that night we were all terrified.
Tommy started to have a go at him and my other brother
Brian stepped in to try to calm things down, which luckily
he managed to do. It was awful.

We never really talked about those incidents afterwards. They were swept under the carpet. We'd just go
to bed and get up the next day and act as if nothing
had happened. Don't get me wrong, these fights didn't
happen every day. There would often be weeks or even
months where nothing happened and Dad was happy.
But when he wasn't happy, we learnt to stay out of his
way.

There were a few occasions when I was on the receiving
end of my dad's temper. When the younger girls were

naughty he'd give us a slap, but it was always heavy-handed to be honest. One night, Linda, Coleen and I were playing in our bedroom. Linda and I were messing about, laughing and whispering instead of going to sleep, so my dad came upstairs and stormed into our room.

'Right, I warned you,' he shouted, pulling back the sheets and smacking Linda and me really hard on our legs until we sobbed and pleaded with him to stop.

'Now I'm going to have to smack her as well,' he said, turning to Coleen, who must have only been about four at the time and hadn't been misbehaving at all. I remember thinking then how wrong that was.

'I didn't do anything!' she wailed, but her words fell on deaf ears and he battered her too. We all wet the bed that night because we were too scared to get up and go to the toilet. All of us were frightened of my dad. If I'd done something wrong, he only had to look at me and I'd wet myself from sheer terror.

But although my dad was incredibly stern and unbelievably strict, he did have a good side to him, which is the side I loved. He could be a lot of fun and always made us feel special. Going to the cinema with him was a regular thing – a different one of us would accompany him each week – and he took an interest in our school work, which my mum never had time for. As well as all the drinking and rowing that went on, I also remember lots of joy, laughter and parties, and my dad was always at the centre of the fun.

As I got older I realised he was fighting a battle within himself. He loved his family, but it wasn't the life he would have chosen, being responsible for eight kids and struggling to make ends meet. But it wasn't my mum's fault and it wasn't our fault either.

Dad started taking less and less interest in my mum after Coleen was born. My mum put on a lot of weight when she was pregnant with Coleen and she stopped caring about her appearance. We all told her she was still gorgeous and tried to encourage her to make more of an effort with her looks – not for my dad's benefit, but so she'd feel better about herself. Anne managed to persuade her to lose a bit of weight and she started to wear nail varnish and make-up again. It was lovely to see her regain some of her confidence and self-esteem. A couple of us said to Dad one day, 'Doesn't Mum look great?' And he replied, 'No she looks ill, she looked better the way she was.' It was crushing for my mum, so she just let herself go again. I was only about ten, but I felt heartbroken for her because I could see how much effort she'd made. I don't think Dad was in love with Mum at that point. I'm not sure if he ever was.

Luckily, I was close to my brothers and sisters growing up. Linda and I were particularly close because we're so near in age. We went everywhere together, but whenever Linda had a boyfriend she'd drop me like a ton of bricks. I always took her back though! We fought, as all siblings do, but if anyone was mean to me at school, she'd stick up for me and both of us looked out for Coleen. We had a fight with a boy once because he was bullying Coleen – he never did it again!

I was never quite as close with Anne because she was ten

years older than me and very bossy. She was like a second mum really and tried to help take care of us; but back then I thought she enjoyed bossing us around a little too much. I can't bear being told what to do now and I think it's a reaction to feeling bossed around when I was little. Looking back I wonder if Anne was doing it because my dad had been so strict with her. He was very hard on the older girls, but by the time Linda, Coleen and I came along he was a bit more lenient. Maybe she felt it was unfair.

My dad had a rule that we never worked at Christmas. It was a special time in our house and we looked forward to it for weeks beforehand. Mum used to do a huge grocery shop – you've never seen so much food! Sometimes on Christmas day there would be twenty-six of us squashed around our dining table. Mum was always inviting people at the last minute to come and join us. *The more the merrier* was her motto. So Christmases were always big noisy affairs.

Because there were so many kids, our presents were stacked halfway up the Christmas tree. We each got a big present and lots of little ones too. I don't know how my parents managed to afford it all. I'm sure some of our gifts must have been second-hand, but we were none the wiser.

We had set ways of doing things, like most families. We always had a cooked breakfast on Christmas morning, but we'd open our presents first. When we were really young, we'd get up at 6 a.m., when my parents had only just finished setting them out under the tree! Linda and I both got prams one year, which we adored and spent hours walking around the neighbourhood.

Once we'd opened our presents from Santa, we'd sit in a circle and give presents to each other, while Mum walked around putting the discarded wrapping paper in bin-bags. Then we'd sit round the table and eat a huge breakfast.

After lunch, which was a traditional turkey feast with all the trimmings, we'd sing carols around the table, followed by 'Have Yourself a Merry Little Christmas' and 'White Christmas' in harmony. My mum would do the octave above us because she was a soprano. Then on Christmas night we always had a big party, which inevitably involved lots of drinking, dancing and fun!

Just before Christmas 1973, Dad was asked if we'd perform at the Cliffs Hotel in Blackpool, as a big company from London was having their Christmas do there. The company was called Hanover Grand and the owner was a guy called Joe Lewis, who was an incredibly wealthy business man and a real player in the entertainment world.

'No, absolutely not. We never work at Christmas,' Dad told the club manger. But in the end we were offered so much money, he couldn't turn it down. That was the performance that changed our lives.

Joe loved our act and came up to us after the show and said, 'Look, I've got a club in London, called the London Rooms. It's on Drury Lane and I want the girls to come down and sing there.'

He felt there was more scope for just the girls as opposed to the entire family. His offer came at just the right time, because the older girls were sick of singing in working men's clubs and felt it was time they got proper jobs. If it hadn't been for Joe Lewis seeing potential in us, I'm convinced we'd have given it all up.

We were offered a good wage and the deal was that we'd sing in the restaurant six nights a week. Joe and his wife Esther even offered to put us up at their house in Wentworth, Surrey. We didn't know it then, but he was already grooming us for TV and a recording contract.

Fortunately, my brothers didn't want to come with us. By now, Tommy was twenty-four and Brian was nineteen. They both loved Blackpool and had serious girlfriends who they were engaged to.

But while us girls were thrilled about the idea of moving to London, Dad wasn't sure about Joe's offer, probably because it meant him giving up control of the group and because it was also a big deal for us to move nearly 200 miles away from home. He kept procrastinating, so in the end it was Mum who signed the contract. 'Oh just sign it, for God's sake!' she snapped, grabbing a pen and signing her name. 'If we don't, they'll be hanging around clubs all their lives.' It was Mum's assertiveness that launched us into the next chapter of our lives.

So, with the deal signed, sealed and delivered, The Nolan Sisters packed our bags to move to London, excited about our big new adventure down South. I was thirteen years old.

2
LONDON LIFE

....

I gasped when I saw Joe's Surrey mansion for the first time – to me it looked like a stately home straight out of *Jane Eyre*. It was a world away from our Waterloo Road terrace. It had big iron gates and a long sweeping driveway surrounded by beautiful gardens and lined with huge oak trees.

'My God, we're going to live here?!' I exclaimed, as we walked through the grounds, trying to take in the splendour of our new home from home. I felt like I was in *Alice Through the Looking Glass* as I explored the sprawling property – there were tennis courts, a swimming pool, ten cavernous bedrooms and endless corridors that went off in different directions. I felt like I could disappear in that house, never to be seen again. It was incredible!

You would imagine that Joe's wife Esther wouldn't be too pleased to have six girls and their mother descend on her, but she was so welcoming. I think she was glad of the company. Joe was always working and she seemed pretty lonely. Esther was Irish like us, with fiery red hair and blue eyes. Joe looked pretty flash – he was Jewish with black slick-backed hair and drove a Jag – but he was really nice with it. They had two children – Charlie and Vivienne who were the same ages as Coleen and me. The kids accepted us really well, considering they'd been invaded! We used to have lunch together every Sunday with posh crockery and candelabras on the table, and the maid would serve us.

Coleen wasn't with us all the time. At nine, she was still too young to perform with us full-time and she missed home and going to the stables – she was mad about horse riding. So she went back to Blackpool and came down occasionally to perform. Dad stayed at home most of the time too, but if he came to London to sing, Coleen was taken care of by Mum's sister, Auntie Theresa, and her husband, Uncle Jim.

Esther was so generous – always encouraging us to play tennis or have a swim in the pool. She used to wait up for us to come home from a show – she'd always be sitting in the snooker room on a leather sofa in front of a huge telly with a glass of wine in her hand and she'd always offer the older girls one too. She enjoyed having us there, but we were all really nice well-brought-up girls after all. How could she not?

We loved the Wentworth period – it was a magical time. We were young and ambitious, and desperate to carve out a professional career in the music business. We were just at the start of everything and it was tremendously exciting. Before we had a driver we had to get the train home after gigs. We used to walk home from Virginia

Water station along dark leafy lanes and one of the older girls would pretend to be a bloke, wearing a big overcoat and acting really butch so we wouldn't get accosted! Hilarious.

Unfortunately, our little Wentworth adventure only lasted six months. We needed to get our own house, so Coleen and my dad could join us permanently. Joe found us somewhere in Ilford, Essex. By Waterloo Road standards, our new house was massive. It used to be an old doctor's surgery and before that it was a school. It had big white pillars either side of the front door and we thought it was pretty posh. I didn't know it then, but I would have some of the best times of my life in that house. Dad put a bar in the conservatory, which we called Flannigan's Bar, and we had a lot of parties!

We were sent to a private school at the bottom of our road called Clark's School for Girls. I'll never forget our first day. Linda, Coleen and I were wearing these awful matching dresses and had to stand in front of the entire school while a teacher introduced us as 'the Nolan girls'. Everyone was looking at us like we'd been beamed in from another planet. I don't think they could quite believe what we were wearing. I couldn't wait to get the uniform, so I could blend in. I enjoyed school though, particularly sport, and thought I might be a PE teacher if the singing didn't work out.

In the evenings, we'd ditch our school uniforms for our stage outfits. Even at thirteen I hated our costumes. Joe had brought in a guy called Robert Earl Senior, who managed us for a while. His wife Daphne was charged with sorting out our image and she was the one who decided we all had to dress the same, which was ridiculous because Anne was ten years older than me. She put us in really conservative Jaeger dresses – not the sort of thing you want to wear when you're thirteen. I used to cry when she made us try those hideous things on.

'We'll have no Sarah Bernhardts from you, dear. Just do as you're told,' she'd snap, and I had to do as I was told. But I hated everything I was given to wear and complained constantly. I was always outvoted by the other girls, though, because they said Robert and Daphne knew what they were doing. But those outfits created a really sweet sickly image that we struggled for years to get rid of. I'm not sure we ever did get rid of it.

We hadn't been performing at the London Rooms for long when an important producer called Stewart Morris came to see us. He was also Head of Light Entertainment at the BBC and the next time he showed up he brought Cliff Richard with him. Cliff had a new TV series and Stewart thought The Nolan Sisters would make great guest stars on the show every week. Cliff loved our act – I remember catching a glimpse of him in the audience, waving his serviette in the air and whooping and hollering! A couple of days later we found out we'd been booked to appear on all six of Cliff's shows. We were going to be on telly! None of us could believe it and we were all jumping up and down, screaming with excitement.

Stewart brought in a guy called Alan Ainsworth to help us. He was a brilliant musical director and a lovely guy too. He arranged all our songs and taught us the harmonies.

We also had Nigel Lythgoe – a top choreographer at the time – to devise our dance routines.

We went to Alan's house every day for a couple of weeks before each show to learn the new songs. I'll never forget our first performance on Cliff's show. Our outfits were bloody disgusting – floor-length green dresses that would have looked better hanging from a curtain pole! Even Coleen, who was nine, was wearing one. At least Stewart Morris had the good sense to insist that hers was shortened.

My school friends used to tease me about my stage outfits. 'What are you wearing?' they'd say. 'God, you're such a geek!' Luckily, my shyness had well and truly disappeared by then and I was feisty and outspoken, so I just ignored them. But they were right! If I'd been watching us on telly, I would have hated us too!

The good thing, of course, was that we could all sing and our harmonies were brilliant. We use to do really difficult *a capella* stuff, but I felt we never really got appreciated for that because people were too busy taking the mickey out of our image.

I remember sitting in the make-up chair at the BBC before that first show, feeling so excited and a little over-awed. I couldn't quite believe we were about to be beamed into people's living-rooms across the country.

We sang a song called 'Now I'm Stuck on You', which was written for us by EMI. We released a few records with EMI around the time we started appearing on TV and Bruce Welch from The Shadows used to do a lot of the production. They were good songs, but none of them were hits – in my opinion, it was too hard for people to make the leap from watching these sugary sweet sisters on telly to buying our records. It would be years before we had a hit record.

We appeared on TV a lot after Cliff's series. We did the *Musical Time Machine* with Vince Hill, *The Morecambe & Wise Christmas Show*, *Mike Yarwood's Christmas Show*, *The Two Ronnies* and *The Harry Secombe Show*.

It was an amazing time and we got the chance to meet so many lovely people. We met Olivia Newton-John on Cliff's show and became quite friendly with her. Once she came by our dressingroom and said, 'Would you guys like to come shopping one day?'

'Yeah! We'd love it!' we all replied enthusiastically.

'OK, I'll give you a call.'

Olivia was gorgeous and we all loved her. I remember thinking, 'If I ever make it big in this business, I hope I can stay as lovely as she is.' She was so unaffected and lovely to everyone. She was about twenty-five at the time and probably mostly interested in being friends with Anne and Maureen, but it was lovely that she invited all of us.

True to her word, she called us at our house in Ilford about 9 a.m. one day.

'OK, we're going to go shopping today!' she said. 'Come to Heathrow for about 11. We're going to fly to Paris.'

'WHAT?' I think that's when the penny dropped that we were in a different league to Olivia. There was no way we could afford to fly to Paris at a moment's notice, let alone find the money to go shopping there.

One of the older girls quickly made the excuse that we had to rehearse. We didn't have a lot of money at that point – we were just starting out.

* * *

We carried on singing at the London Rooms alongside all the TV appearances and released more records with EMI, none of which made any impact. Then in 1975 something happened that did help to launch us into the big leagues. Stewart Morris had been asked to suggest support acts for Frank Sinatra's European tour and he put our name forward. We were stunned. Dad was even more shocked. We'd grown up on Sinatra's music, because my dad was such a huge fan. In fact, he'd recently bought two tickets on the black market for the Sinatra show, which cost him £200 – a fortune back then. He was going to have one of the tickets and raffle the other one between the rest of us.

Stewart warned us that Frank's people were looking at four other acts besides us and that Frank himself was going to choose which group got the gig. So when Stewart called to tell us we were on the tour, we were totally blown away. It felt like all our birthdays and Christmases had come at once. We were running through our house in Ilford, screaming – all six of us!

Sinatra had a sixty-piece orchestra, which we were allowed to use. For our opening night, at the Palais des Congrès in Paris, we brought along Alan Ainsworth as our musical director. We'd put a whole new set together and couldn't wait to try it out in front of an audience.

I'd come down with a bad cold though, and coughed all the way through an *a capella* version of a song called 'Scarlet Ribbons'. I sounded like a dog barking, and of course the French audience all laughed. It was truly awful. I was only fifteen and I came straight off stage and cried my eyes out. It was also the night we were going to be introduced to Mr Sinatra.

As we walked down the corridor to meet him, I could hear his voice and felt so nervous. Can you imagine being introduced to Frank Sinatra?

'Oh, hi,' he said when he saw us, reaching out to shake our hands. 'So which one of you kids has got a cough?'

Oh God, here we go, I thought. 'Um, that'll be me,' I said sheepishly.

'Hey, don't you worry about it, honey. It's all good experience.'

He couldn't have been nicer to us. And he was right – those kinds of experiences help you grow as a performer.

On that tour we got to see every soundcheck and every show for two weeks. At the soundcheck Sinatra would come over to us and sing a song, and say things like, 'You kids won't know this one.' Of course we wanted to say, 'We do know them all! We love you!' But we didn't want to sound gushing, so we didn't say anything at all!

One of the best things was being able to introduce Sinatra to my dad when we played the Royal Albert Hall in London.

'Mr Sinatra, this is our dad,' we said.

'Hi Mr Nolan, you must be so proud of your daughters,' Frank replied, shaking Dad's hand.

But Dad was so stunned at being face to face with his hero that he couldn't speak. He just mumbled, 'Beautiful. Beautiful.'

'Dad!' I said, digging him in the ribs. Usually, he was a very eloquent man, but he was completely overwhelmed to be in Frank's presence. I think he was deeply touched by it. I almost expected him to cry.

Afterwards, though, he was like an excited little boy.

Years later, after my dad had died, I was very grateful we'd been able to do that for him. It was the greatest gift we could have given him.

At the end of the tour, Frank gave each of us a gold key ring, engraved with the words, 'Love and peace, Frank Sinatra.'

What the hell were we going to buy Frank Sinatra? His daughter Nancy had just had a baby, AJ, so we decided to buy a beautiful life-size doll for her and we gave it to Frank's PA to pass on to him.

On our last night in Belgium we were standing at our dressingroom door, ready to go and watch the show, when we saw Sinatra walking down the corridor with Elizabeth Taylor, who looked unbelievably glamorous – a proper old-school movie star. They were totally surrounded by journalists and photographers.

'Excuse me for a sec, Liz,' said Sinatra. Then he turned to the press pack. 'Can you let me through, guys? There's something I've gotta do.'

He started walking towards us and I looked at my sisters and whispered, 'Oh my God, what have we done?' under my breath.

'Guys, thank you so much for the doll,' he said, breaking into a huge grin. 'AJ's gonna love that. It was a beautiful thought.'

'You're welcome!' we all said in unison, sounding like a bunch of idiots.

What an experience for a fifteen-year-old girl! At the time, I probably didn't really appreciate the opportunity we'd been given, but looking back it was nothing short of amazing. Sinatra had so much charisma on stage. As well as being a sensational singer, he knew the importance of putting on a performance and being able to talk to the audience. And that's something we all learnt from him during that tour.

Considering we were together 24/7, living and working with each other, us girls got along pretty well. Maureen was so easy-going anyway – really gentle with a sweet and caring nature. And she was beautiful. She was the Nolan all the boys made a beeline for! Linda was very strong-minded and gobby – she was probably the only one of us who wasn't scared to stand up to my dad. After a show at the London Rooms, she'd often call Dad at home and say, 'I'm going out, Dad.'

'No you're not. Get back here!' he'd reply.

'Yes, we are going out. See ya later,' she'd chirp, before hanging up. The rest of us wouldn't have dared to talk to Dad like that.

Coleen was the baby, of course, so we all looked out for her, and I was pretty feisty and opinionated. I clashed a bit with Denise because she was so much older, and I was usually at loggerheads with Anne because we both had fiery tempers. I'd always resented her bossiness as a kid, then when I got into my teens it felt like she was always trying to embarrass me in front of boys I fancied.

When we first moved to our house in Ilford, there was a guitar player I really liked. It was just puppy love because I was only a kid and he was much older than I was. Sometimes he'd come back to our house after the show and Anne would make a point of saying, 'Little girls should be seen and not heard. Get up to bed.' I felt she made a show of me in front of him. I used to go to bed and cry, 'I hate her! I hate her!'

Then when I was sixteen I started dating a really handsome Turkish guy I'd met at the London Rooms, who was four years older than I was. I guess he was my first big crush. There was never any question that we'd have a physical relationship – I was quite innocent back then! – but he took me to London for the day and I bought new jeans especially for the date. We had a kiss and it was very sweet.

I was too young to go for a drink after our shows at the London Rooms, but Anne would go and she hung out with this guy I'd been seeing. I was friendly with a woman who worked on the door and one night she said to me, 'Your Anne was here last night, smooching on the dance floor with your guy and kissing him.'

I felt totally heartbroken. I was only a kid but I'd already been out with him. In the end, it all came to a head and we had a massive fight.

The fight started when we were getting ready for our show one night and Anne had rollers in her hair. I yanked them out without taking the clips out first and she hit me across the face. I thought, 'Right, I'm sixteen now, I'm not standing for this any more,' and I whacked her back. She couldn't believe it. In the past, I'd never have retaliated if she'd given me a slap.

We always laugh about the fight now because it was so crazy. Anne jumped on my back and ripped my jumper and I pulled her hair. I guess it was quite good, in a way, because it got years of pent-up frustration out of my system and it never happened again.

With hindsight I can see why Anne felt the way she did. She'd never been allowed to have any freedom and now she could see Linda and me having boyfriends and going out and having fun. My dad was definitely more lenient with the younger girls, and I suspect Anne felt angry about that and a bit jealous. I don't think she was even allowed to mention boys till she was about twenty-three, let alone date them. There was also a far more sinister subtext to Anne's relationship with my dad, which didn't emerge until many years later after Dad had died. But at that point, we didn't understand why Anne seemed to be angry.

We loved singing at the London Rooms – it was great regular work – but every time we released a record with EMI it flopped. I frequently used to think, 'Oh God we're never gonna do it!' And I was convinced that we'd never be properly accepted with our 'holier than thou' image, even if we could sing bloody well. In my opinion no one sang harmonies as well as us at the time, so it was really frustrating. We were household names because of all the telly we'd done, but we still couldn't get that elusive hit record.

Then in 1977 we were offered a deal performing on a cruise ship called the *Orsova*. I'd left school the year before, after my O-levels, to put everything into the group. We might not have made it on to *Top of the Pops* yet, but singing was still my passion in life and I was determined to keep going.

My dad accompanied us on the cruise as our manager and chaperone.

One night he came down to the cabin and said, 'I've met this guy in the bar who's perfect for you. He's from an Irish family in Derby. Come and meet him; he's in the bar upstairs.'

I literally couldn't believe what I was hearing. My dad had been terrifyingly strict when I was a kid, which I honestly think scarred the older girls for life. But although he'd definitely mellowed with age and allowed me to have more freedom, I still wasn't expecting him to say something like that!

I couldn't explain it, but I suppose as I got into my later teens Dad and I had a certain rapport. We both loved Sinatra and big band music, and jazz, and we both liked to drink and socialise. I think I have some qualities that my dad lacked, and I later came to realise he was very misguided, but in some ways we were similar.

But I couldn't imagine what this guy was like if my dad thought he was a good match for me. I expected him to be vile, but I agreed to go up to the ship's Monkey Bar to meet him anyway. He was called Mike Callahan and, to my utter surprise and delight, he was drop-dead gorgeous!

He had thick jet-black hair, big blue eyes and a gorgeous tan because he'd been on the ship for ages. I fell for him hook, line and sinker!

He was head barman, although he was only eighteen, and used to do all those fancy moves when he was making cocktails, which I was so impressed by!

We arranged to go on a date when the ship docked in Barbados – he'd been there lots of times before and offered to show me the sights. On the day of our date, the whole family decided to go on this little cruise around

Barbados called 'the Jolly Roger', which was brilliant fun. They played Caribbean music and the rum cocktails flowed all day, and we dived off the boat into the crystal clear sea.

But I got absolutely hammered on the cocktails. Looking back, it's probably the most drunk I've ever been in my life. Being a teenager, I didn't know when to stop. When we got back to the ship, I crawled into my bunk, feeling like death.

'You've got your date. You can't stay in bed!' said Linda. 'Have a sleep, but you've only got three hours, then you'll have to get up and have a shower. OK?'

'I'm not going,' I mumbled, burying my head in the pillow.

'Oh yes, you are going,' she replied sternly. 'You really like him and he's gorgeous!'

I went to sleep, but three hours later Linda couldn't wake me up, so she lifted me out of bed, carried me into the shower and threw me under a jet of cold water, fully clothed. Well, that woke me up! She then helped me to get dressed and poured loads of black coffee down my neck. Eventually, I did sober up in time to go on my date with Mike and I was glad of Linda's act of sisterly love!

Mike and I had a wonderful night. Some of his friends from the ship came along and we visited some of the famous bars, then went for a meal.

As first dates go, it was pretty perfect. Mike and I walked back to the ship alone and had a kiss. It was a beautiful balmy evening, the Caribbean sea was glistening, palm trees were silhouetted against the night sky and you could hear steel drums in the distance. It really

was incredibly romantic. I'll never forget those first feelings of love and passion – it was one of the best moments
of my life.

As well as being very handsome, Mike was also a lovely
guy. We saw each other for the rest of the time we spent
on the ship and when the cruise was over I cried when
we had to part. However, I was going on a UK tour with
The Nolan Sisters soon, and we were going to be in Derby,
so Mike asked me to come and stay with him and his
mum for a night.

I'd just turned eighteen and was still a virgin when I
visited Mike in Derby. We'd been writing letters to each
other since the cruise and we couldn't wait to see each
other. When I got to his mum's house, he said, 'I'll take
your case upstairs.' So I followed him up. 'This is
where we're sleeping,' he said casually, dumping my bag
on the double bed. Er, *we're* sleeping! I nearly dropped
dead on the spot. Looking back, it was very cheeky of
him to assume we were going to share a bed – he really
should have given me a choice!

That night when we got into bed I was dying with
embarrassment because when it came to boys I was quite
shy. I'd never slept with anyone, and up until this point
Mike and I had only kissed. My sisters were the only
people who'd seen me naked!

I went to the bathroom to get undressed, then quickly
jumped into bed in my very unsexy pyjamas, pulling the
sheets up underneath my chin. Then Mike came back
from the bathroom with just his boxers on. I remember
thinking, 'Wow!' because he had such a great body and
was still tanned from the cruise. I was so embarrassed

and nervous that I blurted out, 'Oh! You're just in your boxer shorts then?' God, I felt like such a fool.

Mike started to kiss me and one thing led to another. He was so lovely and gentle. As first experiences go, I couldn't have imagined anything better. It was beautiful. I was ready to do it and it was wonderful that it happened with someone I really cared about and who cared about me too.

I felt so embarrassed facing his mum at breakfast the next day, but she was lovely. 'Morning!' she chirped as I walked into the kitchen.

'Ahem, morning,' I replied sheepishly.

I had to do the show that night, then Mike had to go back to the ship, so we said our goodbyes.

'I'll see you soon,' he said, taking my hand. 'I'm crazy about you . . . I love you.'

I didn't quite know what to say to that. 'Er, I'm mad about you too,' I said, blushing.

I told my sisters I'd lost my virginity and they were so excited for me, although I'm sure some of them were still virgins at the time! None of us were very experienced, to be honest.

Mike and I went back to writing to each other and had phone calls when we could. We dated for about a year, but I hardly ever saw him because he worked on the ship and things just petered out. We were still so young.

In 1978 Denise decided to leave the group to become a solo artist, which I think was the right choice for her. She enjoyed singing, but she hated the choreography and she didn't feel she fitted in. Plus she was twenty-six and was in a serious relationship with her boyfriend Tom. That same year we made an album called *20 Giant Hits*, with Warner Bros, which Denise had also sung on. It was an album of cover versions and it sold like hotcakes, getting to number three in the charts. We were all stunned that it was such a success – we got a gold disc for it.

All of a sudden, the huge record companies were courting us because we'd sold so many records – not just EMI and Warner Bros, but also CBS. We decided to go for CBS and they employed respected songwriters Ben Findon and Mike Myers to write for us.

At the start of 1979, we went into the studio to hear a ballad they'd penned for us called 'Spirit, Body and Soul', which I loved. When we started recording it, each of us had to have a go at singing the lead vocal and I was picked.

It was our first single with CBS and it got to number thirty-four in the charts. Our A&R guy, Nicky Graham, called to give us the good news. 'Oh, and you'll be doing *Top of the Pops* on Thursday,' he added. 'You're going to be huge!'

Singing on that show had been a childhood dream and I was about to fulfil it. It was finally happening.

3
WE'VE MADE IT!

....

As we walked out of our dressingroom at the BBC to make our way to the *Top of the Pops* studio, we bumped right into Scottish punk band The Skids. 'Urrgh, The Nolans,' said the lead singer Richard Jobson, spitting on the floor by our feet. 'Wow, welcome to *Top of the Pops*!' I thought.

Punk was still around and here we were, making our debut on the show, looking so prim in our sweet dresses. Some of those bands were really nasty to us and we took a lot of crap from them, but I guess we must have seemed really out of place and old-fashioned.

At least our dresses were different colours on this occasion, so we were expressing some individuality, but they were still vile. I was nineteen by now and well and truly sick of being told what to wear.

Robert and his wife Daphne had been kicked into touch long ago, but Stewart Morris, who sometimes directed *Top of the Pops*, was still keen to portray a certain image of us.

'Look, I'll decide what you wear on the show,' he said when I complained for the umpteenth time.

'You're not in charge of us any more,' I said. 'We're young girls and we want to wear what's fashionable now, like jeans!'

So finally, after years of complaining about our stage outfits, we got to wear drainpipe jeans. We still had to wear the same shirt in different colours to keep a theme, but at least our image was a bit more modern, and we gradually started wearing clothes we wanted to wear. I was delighted!

At the time we were one of the few acts that sang live on *Top of the Pops*, which had a live BBC orchestra in the studio. All the punk bands got away with miming, but the show had to have a certain number of groups singing live and we were always one of them. So no matter how good we sounded – and we did sound great live – the production values on the other songs were always much better because they just played the record!

I hated the next song Mike and Ben wrote for us – 'I'm in the Mood for Dancing'. It was really poppy and jangly and not my cup of tea at all. I was listening to Chaka Khan, Stevie Wonder and lots of blues, soul and jazz music. 'Oh, I really don't like that,' I said, turning my nose up, when they played it to us in the studio. '"I'm in the mood for dancing" is such a cheesy line. I hate it!'

'But this is commercial, Bernie, it's going to work. Go with it,' advised Ben. The other girls liked it too, so I was outvoted. And of course it shot to number three in the singles chart where it stayed for sixteen weeks and was our biggest hit ever! And it made number one in lots of other countries around the world.

'Take that, Richard Jobson!' I thought to myself. 'You can sod off!'

It really was a great, great feeling to have that kind of success. I was buzzing. Our *Top of the Pops* performances for that song were much better, too. Of course, now we were wearing jeans – thank God – and although we were still singing live, we could sing to a backing track of our own music rather than the BBC orchestra. Don't get me wrong, those musicians were all brilliant, but they could never replicate the sound of our record – we had guitars, while they had bloody strings and a full brass section!

Top of the Pops became a pretty regular thing after that. Between 1979 and 1983 we had twelve top twenty hits in a row, including 'Don't Make Waves', 'Gotta Pull Myself Together', 'Attention to Me', 'Who's Gonna Rock You?' and 'Chemistry'. We were on the bill with some great acts – Kim Wilde, and Bonnie Tyler with her monster hit, 'Total Eclipse of the Heart'.

In 1980 Anne left the group. She'd recently married her boyfriend, Brian Wilson, who was a professional footballer with Blackpool, and wanted to settle into married life, so Coleen took her place. Up until that point, Coleen had only been a part-time member, joining us for occasional performances, and she hadn't sung on 'I'm in the Mood for Dancing'. Our success meant the record company had major tours planned for us so, with our revamped line-up, we shortened our name to The Nolans – rather than The Nolan Sisters – and prepared to take the world by storm. First stop was a promotional tour of Japan, where we were massive. When we got off the plane it was like The

Beatles had arrived – there was a huge crowd of screaming fans to greet us, all shouting our names and waving banners. It was nuts.

We couldn't leave our hotel room without causing a stampede. I got punched in the nose by a fan who was trying to grab me as I left a gig. We had to have police escorts to and from the venues. Looking back it was brilliant, but at the time it was pretty scary. I remember thinking, 'Jesus, what's it like to be Michael Jackson?' I wasn't sure I was comfortable with all that attention because it was impossible to do normal things. And it was a bit boring to be honest, because when we weren't working we were holed up in our hotel room to avoid being mobbed.

And I missed my boyfriend Bob terribly – phone calls and letters were a poor substitute for being together. We'd started dating the year before after meeting at a bar in Ilford called the Villa. I used to go there on a Saturday with my cousin Angie, who was living with us at the time. I saw him staring at me from across the bar and I'd just said to Angie, 'Ooh, he's nice,' when he got up from his seat and walked over to us and introduced himself. His name was Bob Allison and he was a car salesman from Essex. We ended up spending the whole evening together and we began dating after that. He had dark hair like Mike and was very kind and funny.

I also struggled with the food in Japan. Sometimes our days were so packed with newspaper and radio interviews, they didn't schedule any time for us to eat and we'd have to explain that we were hungry. Then one of the runners would usually go out and bring back sushi, which we all hated.

Linda's boyfriend Brian Hudson – who she married the following year – was our tour manager at the time, so he'd often go on a hunt for burgers. The rest of the time we lived on plain rice. Luckily, my mum had also brought a load of English tea bags and biccies with her!

One day we were invited to a green tea ceremony with a monk who offered us these tiny biscuits to eat and they were probably the worst things I've ever tasted in my life. But it would have been so insulting to spit them out, so we all swallowed hard, even though we wanted to vomit!

Later that year we went back to Japan for the Tokyo Music Festival, which is their version of the Eurovision Song Contest, and played alongside people like Randy Crawford and Jermaine Jackson. We ended up winning it, becoming the first European act ever to take top prize. Our popularity was mind-boggling really – we sold nine million records in Japan alone. Whenever we played, people threw presents on stage for us and we'd have to duck to avoid getting felled by a flying umbrella or a stuffed toy. One time, Linda got knocked out on stage by a watch and we had to drag her into the wings. We ended up sending hundreds of cuddly toys back to children's homes in the UK.

We travelled to other countries around the world, too – I loved Australia particularly – but Japan was the place we visited most often. In 1981 we returned for a proper tour with our band and we got to see more of the country and enjoy ourselves a bit more, too. We used to play cards between shows with the guys in the band and we got to ride the bullet train, which we loved. One night we played the Budokan, which is the biggest venue in Tokyo, but there was a power cut so all the lights and sound went off and we ended up going on stage with torches under our chins, singing *a capella* to 15,000 people until they fixed the problem – and the audience loved it.

Back in glamorous Ilford, my twenty-first birthday was coming up and I'd planned a big fancy-dress party at our house. There were relatives coming over from Dublin and loads of my friends from Essex. I'd made lots of great friends through Bob, who was a local lad. There were about thirteen couples and we had this 'no solids on a Sunday' rule where we'd go to the pub and just drink all day! More often than not, we'd all pile back to Bob's place in Barkingside or to my parents' house and grab a pizza on the way. We were all young and in love, and we had a really great laugh together.

On the morning of my twenty-first, my mum and dad popped their heads around my bedroom door and said, 'Can you come outside for a minute?' When I got downstairs all my sisters and brothers were there and they were all telling me to go outside. 'Go on, Bernie. Go and have a look!' they were saying.

So I opened the front door and on the driveway was my first car – a green Mini with L-plates on it and a huge bow. 'Happy birthday!' everyone shouted. Bob had got Mum and Dad a good deal on the car and I was beyond thrilled with it.

Later in the day everyone started arriving in fancy dress. One of my mates – a 6ft black guy called Laurie – turned up dressed as a baby, which was just about the funniest thing I'd ever seen. I went as Wonder Woman and stuffed my bra with knickers to boost my cleavage. My brother Brian went as Noddy, and the bell on his hat kept ringing while he was trying to chat up my best friend Julie Davy.

'Yeah, very sexy, Brian. I love yer bell!' I said as I passed them in the hallway.

And my Auntie Phyllis and Uncle Peter came as Cleopatra and Julius Caesar, wearing short togas. He was a boxer and had won a bronze medal at the Olympics. He had to keep his cigarettes in his underpants because there were no pockets in his toga! Linda and her husband came as clowns and their costumes were so good, none of us realised who they were for about half an hour. And Auntie Lily, who was in her late eighties by then, came as a punk rocker – complete with fake safety pin through her nose, ripped fishnets and a mini skirt. She looked hysterically funny.

My dad was behind the bar, serving drinks, and Mum had made loads of food. And, of course, there was lots of music and dancing. It was one of the best days of my life – everyone still talks about what a great party it was. Fancy dress is a wonderful icebreaker.

After my twenty-first, I moved in with Bob in Barkingside, which is only up the road from Ilford, so I could go to and from Bob's and my parents' house in my little Mini. It was a funny existence though, because he had a normal nine-to-five job and I'd often have to work at night or go away on tour.

We were playing the cabaret circuit by then, which meant going on stage at 11 p.m. Linda and I used to share hotel rooms and go to sleep listening to Radio 2 after a sandwich and a cup of tea. That kind of good behaviour didn't last long, though!

We also did major UK tours a couple of times a year, playing big theatres like the Dominion in London's Tottenham Court Road and the Odeon in Birmingham, which is no longer there. For the first time, we had our own sound and lighting rig, and our own band called Car Park. Robin Smith was the MD and he went on to work with Chaka Khan. Phil Cranham played bass, Paul Donnelly was on guitar and Dave Early, who was our drummer, went on to play for Sade. Very sadly, he died in a car crash and Mel Gaynor became our drummer, and he later played with Simple Minds. They were all brilliant musicians.

On tour we were able to put funkier tracks into the set list, as well as our back catalogue, so it was fun and very different to what people had seen us do on telly. We had lasers and smoke and a really big sound – it was such an exciting time. I was in my element.

We also travelled in a luxury tour bus and had lots of laughs on the road. I got on well with my sisters most of the time, although I had very definite opinions about music – I was into black American soul and hated schmaltzy pop with a passion! When we had to make a decision about the group, Linda and I agreed most of the time, Coleen was always pretty apathetic and tended to go with the flow, which was annoying when we had to vote on something – we wanted her opinion and she didn't have one! Anne and I still clashed – about music and other things too. Our moral compasses were so different. I swore quite a lot and I liked to party! I was probably smoking forty cigarettes and drinking a bottle of vodka or Bacardi a day at this point. I wasn't addicted to booze – I just liked it a lot. It wasn't that Anne was a prude, but we were just very different personalities and those differences got blown up because we were spending every minute of the day with each other.

I used to get into trouble with the other girls – and particularly Anne – for partying too hard. They said I should be looking after my voice because I sang most of the lead vocals. But I was young and just wanted to have a good time. Plus, I think part of the reason I smoked and drank so much was to relieve the pressure of doing so much of the singing.

I suppose I took after my dad when it came to that kind of thing. Officially, I started smoking at eighteen, but really I had my first cigarette when I was just eleven. And as soon as I could drink legally in bars, I did. I remember saying to Dad, 'Look, I drink, you know. I drink Bacardi and Coke.'

'OK then,' was all he said. I couldn't believe he wasn't annoyed about it.

We used to go on stage about 9 p.m., then when we finished a couple of hours later I was full of adrenaline and the last thing I wanted to do was go to bed. I wouldn't have been able to sleep. So I used to stay up until six or seven in the morning, while the rest of the girls and the band went to bed. Even the crew, who had a reputation for partying, couldn't keep up with me.

'You boring old farts,' I'd say, as they drifted off to bed at 4 a.m.

'Bernie, we've got to leave for Glasgow first thing in the morning!' they'd protest.

I'd often stay up talking to the night porter in the hotel, but I always made sure my bag was packed and sitting by the door, so all I had to do was fall out of bed, put my dark glasses on and get on the bus, where I'd fall asleep across the back seats. Everyone knew not to speak to me until at least midday!

I suppose I was quite wild. I smoked joints pretty much every night with the band and the crew, but I was only doing what a lot of other people my age were doing. And I drew the line at harder drugs. A lot of my friends back in Essex were on cocaine, but I never took it. Marijuana just made me laugh a lot, but I never liked the idea of coke – I'd seen how people behaved on it and how addictive it could be, and it wasn't for me.

Towards the end of 1982, Anne rejoined the group and we released a compilation album called *Altogether*, which got to number 52 – disappointing considering our album the year before, *Portrait*, charted at number seven. The single from *Altogether* – 'Dragonfly' – was also a flop and failed to chart at all, and the following year we split with our record company CBS over creative differences. Even though we loved Mike Myers and Ben Findon, we wanted to change our writers to be a bit funkier, but the record company didn't want to take us in that direction.

After that lots of things started to change for The Nolans. We never signed another record deal or had another hit. And, without the support of a giant like CBS behind us, our popularity dwindled – at least in the UK – and we started making less money too.

That same year, Linda left the band. Her husband Brian had been our tour manager, but it wasn't working out. Brian was a great guy and a good tour manager, but he was Linda's husband first and foremost. The rest of us became a bit paranoid that he put her interests first, to the point where we even suspected her mic was louder – crazy stuff like that! He had too much involvement really.

And it was hard for the rest of us to criticise Brian because Linda would get upset. We couldn't be honest about things. It was awkward. Part of a tour manager's job is to take flak from the band, but we didn't feel comfortable doing that with Brian, so it just didn't work. When Brian left, Linda left too – I guess she felt she didn't want to be part of it any more if Brian wasn't involved.

Linda and I weren't as close after that and none of us saw her very much. She became a solo artist, managed by Brian, and put all her energy into their life together. I missed her a great deal, but things in the group were easier in some ways because we weren't arguing so much.

My brother Brian stepped in to become our tour manager and we had some very memorable trips with him. We did a tour of Russia in 1986, playing 25,000-seater stadiums. It was just before the reforms of Perestroika, so there was barely any food, although there was plenty of vodka! Bizarrely, we had caviar and boiled eggs for breakfast. The first hotel we got to in Moscow was filthy and had bloodstained sheets, so Coleen and I refused to stay. The promoter was clearly trying to save money!

We ended up finding a lovely hotel where I celebrated my twenty-sixth birthday. The crew brought some speakers up to the bedroom and we started to party. It wasn't long before one of the hotel guards knocked on the door, though – an incredibly fat stony-faced woman.

'You will not have party here,' she barked.

'Well, it's my birthday, so we are having a party, but we won't cause any problems,' I replied, smiling.

She left and we carried on partying, but ten minutes later there was another loud knock at the door and this time she was accompanied by a soldier in Soviet uniform carrying a machine-gun, which he pointed straight at us.

'You will not have party,' she repeated.

'Er, OK, we will not have party. Night night!'

As well as all the changes in the group, my personal life was changing too. I'd been with Bob for six years, but things had been petering out for a while. As soon as I'd moved in with him I was off on tour, sometimes for six weeks at a time. I was barely at home. It's hard to sustain a relationship in those circumstances, but Bob was so loyal and loving, and such a great guy, that we kept going. We even got engaged – well sort of – one Christmas. He gave me a ring as a present and I said, 'Oh! A ring. Which finger should I put it on?'

'Well, the third finger on your left hand, I would imagine,' he replied. Bob was so laid-back! At the time, though, it wasn't what I wanted. I wanted to be swept off my feet and he wasn't that sort of person. I suppose everything else in my life was quite exciting for most of the time we were dating – hit records and tours – then I'd come home and things would seem so mundane. Bob would be doing his nine-to-five and we'd go to the pub at night. It sounds really immature now, but I guess I was young and I thought the grass was greener. I felt like I was missing out on something – and someone else had also caught my eye.

When I was still with Bob, Coleen started dating our drummer, a guy called Gavin. He was so funny and talented – talent is such a turn-on for me – and I remember thinking how lovely he was. We got on really well together. We were on the same wavelength and liked similar music. Before he started seeing Coleen he used to flirt with me, but I thought 'I'd better nip this in the bud,' because I was with Bob. One day we were at a studio in Hertfordshire rehearsing for a tour and he asked me for my car keys because my car was blocking him in. So he moved it for me and, as I was leaving that night, he said, 'I've put a song on a cassette and left it in your car for you, so you can listen to it on your way home.' The track was 'Suddenly' by Billy Ocean, which is a very romantic song. It was exactly the sort of thing I was looking for from Bob – romance.

When I saw Gavin at rehearsals the next day, I called him over and said, 'Look, what you did was lovely and very touching, but I'm going out with someone.'

After I made it clear I was still happy with Bob, Gavin started seeing Coleen and they ended up going out together for a couple of years.

Then towards the end of their relationship we were on

tour in Dublin and Gavin knocked on my bedroom door one night and said, 'Do you want to go for a walk?' Now I should have said no, because you don't do that when someone is going out with your sister, but I was awake, so I said, 'Yeah.' We'd always got along well as mates, so I told myself it was harmless. Gavin wasn't traditionally handsome – he was very tall and skinny – but he was charismatic and very funny.

We walked around the streets of Dublin in the rain for a while, but nothing happened – we didn't kiss or hold hands. We were attracted to each other though, and we had been flirting. I kept saying to him that if he had strong feelings for anyone other than Coleen, then he needed to tell her. When we got back to the hotel he went off to his room and I went to mine. As I passed Coleen's room, I heard her crying. I wondered if they'd had a row or if he'd come back and told her he'd been for a walk with me, but she never mentioned it.

I felt terrible hearing her upset, though. It was horrendous. Not long afterwards Coleen and Gavin split up and I split up with Bob. I think Gavin made me realise that if I could have such strong feelings for another guy, then I shouldn't be with Bob. And it wasn't fair on Bob either. He was heartbroken and refused to speak to me for a couple of years, but I realised later that he'd done the right thing. It's impossible to get over someone if you keep in touch straight away. We're good friends now, though, and he's happily married with a daughter.

In 1986, The Nolans were booked for a summer season in Bournemouth with Cannon & Ball. A couple of months before the show kicked off, Gavin called me and asked if I'd go out with him.

'Um, I'm not sure about that. It might be awkward,' I said.

'Well, we're both single . . .'

That was true, but Coleen was still upset about the break-up. We did start seeing each other before that summer season but I didn't want to go public with our relationship until Coleen had met someone else. And we were still touring together, which I felt would be harder for her if she knew we were dating.

But when we got to Bournemouth, it all came out. Coleen had met Shane Richie, who she was crazy about and later married, so I decided to tell Maureen I'd been seeing Gavin and hoped she'd break the news to Coleen. I wasn't being cowardly – I genuinely thought she would take it better from Maureen than from me.

Maureen did tell Coleen and when I went into work that night, all she said was, 'Maureen's told me. I don't want to talk about it. It's fine.' I respected her wishes and we never spoke about it again.

Gavin and I were together for three years and lived with each other in his flat in Watford. It was bliss and I really loved him – I just wish he hadn't been my sister's fella. At first it was awkward and I felt uncomfortable at family dos when we were all in a room together, but Coleen was in love with Shane by then, so it worked out OK in the end.

As well as gigging with The Nolans, I started to do a bit of TV presenting. I had more time on my hands now we weren't doing major tours or promoting records. I'd been a guest presenter on kids' show *Cheggers Plays Pop*, presented by Keith Chegwin. The producer was a guy called Martin Hughes and we got on really well. The kids used to love me and I did quite a good job, so I kept getting asked back. I think it was because I used to chuck myself into the games and didn't mind getting covered in foam. I wasn't scared of getting messy! Then in 1988 I got a call from my agent Tony Clayman, saying that Martin had been in touch about me being one of the presenters on a new Saturday morning kids' show called *On the Waterfront*, so I filmed the pilot and ended up presenting the show alongside Kate Copstick, Terry Randall and Andrew O'Connor. We filmed it in the Albert Dock in Liverpool and rehearsed at the BBC in Manchester. I had an absolute ball on that show. I was in charge of the kids' games and we also did sketches every week, which is how I discovered I could act and had good comic timing. We did this skit called 'The Flashing Blade', where we dubbed over an old foreign series. The script was written by Russell T. Davies, who went on to write *Dr Who*. It was hilarious and way ahead of its time. We had so much fun doing it – I used to slide down the walls laughing as we matched our voices to the characters on screen. The show was a big success, so a second series was commissioned.

I was also offered my first panto that year, playing Maid Marion in *Babes in the Wood* at the Palace Theatre in Manchester alongside my old mates Cannon & Ball. And I was approached by EMI to record my own album. To this day, I can't believe I didn't do it. The reason I turned it down was out of loyalty to the other girls in the group. Plus I was busy with *On the Waterfront* and had the panto coming up. Looking back, though, I wish I'd left The Nolans then and tried to make it as a solo artist. Who knows what would have happened? It was a major missed opportunity.

But I was starting to spread my wings and branch into new areas. I was laying the foundations of a career away from my sisters.

4

LOVE AND MARRIAGE

....

'I don't think I love you, Bernie,' said Gavin, who was lying next to me in bed at his flat in Watford, staring up at the ceiling.

'Oh, good morning to you, too!' I replied, throwing the duvet back and jumping out of bed to get dressed. We'd had a huge row the night before and it was obvious our relationship had seen its best days.

We were always arguing because Gavin was absolutely besotted with his drum kit – he practised five hours a day, every day of the week, and we were living in a pretty small flat. I respected the fact that he was so devoted to his craft, but it was hell to live with!

I'd been dividing my time between his place and my mate Dee's house in Blackpool, which was a handy base for work, and I suppose Gavin and I had become friends with benefits rather than boyfriend and girlfriend. The romance and intimacy had gone and, to be frank, we were just using each other for sex. So when he admitted how he felt that morning, I packed my bags and headed back to Blackpool. Although I was upset about breaking up with Gavin, I knew the relationship wasn't right.

I settled back into life in Blackpool and, after living with Dee for a while, I rented a house for myself in Bispham. I wasn't looking for a boyfriend, but my friends and my sisters kept passing messages on to me from a guy called Bradley Walsh. 'Bradley sends his love,' they'd tease.

'Who the hell is this Bradley Walsh character?' I asked Maureen.

'He's an up-and-coming comedian,' she explained. 'But he was a professional footballer. And he's very good-looking.'

'Hmm, is he now?'

That year – 1989 – The Nolans were offered a summer season at the Grand Theatre in Blackpool with The Grumbleweeds. One night before the show, Maureen and Coleen came running into the dressingroom, very excited because they'd just bumped into Bradley Walsh, who had his own show at the Horseshoe Bar.

'Oh my God, he's gorgeous, Bernie!' said Coleen. 'He's got lovely blue eyes and he had a cream rain mac on and he said "Give my love to Bernie. I'm mad about your sister."'

Apparently Coleen and Maureen said, 'But you don't even know Bernie!'

'I know, but I'm crazy about her,' was his reply.

Coleen's boyfriend Shane knew Bradley quite well, as they'd done a TV show together.

'Bradley wants you to come to the Horseshoe and see his show,' said Shane one day. 'So me and Col will take you one night after your show if you like.'

I was a bit nervous, to be honest, because I thought, 'If he's crap I won't fancy him.' For me, talent is an aphrodisiac so if someone isn't good at what they do I find it very off-putting – however good-looking they are!

So one night, we did go to see him perform at the Horseshoe and he was hysterically funny and bloody gorgeous too! We met in the bar afterwards and chatted all night. We hit it off straight away and I could tell that he did really like me.

Soon afterwards a single red rose was delivered to the theatre with a card from Bradley that read: 'You know how I feel . . . let's do dinner.' Oh my God! It was the most romantic thing ever. It was exactly what I'd been looking for with Bob and Gavin. The next thing that happened was that Bradley turned up at the stage door and asked me out. He seemed besotted and I definitely enjoyed being swept off my feet.

I had such a heavenly time that summer. We used to go up to the Lake District and have picnics. Brad is a great singer and we'd lie in the grass on the mountainside while he sang Sinatra and Nat King Cole songs, then we'd laugh until we cried. I was absolutely crazy about him.

His permanent base was a place called Abbots Langley, just outside Watford, so when the summer season was over, I'd flit between his cottage and my place in Blackpool. It was an exciting time. The sex was wonderful, too – we were very compatible physically and that side of things was an important part of the relationship. Maybe I should have realised it was too good to be true.

The following summer I was doing a summer season in Yarmouth with The Nolans and Brad was back at the

Horseshoe in Blackpool with his show when a friend of mine saw him getting really friendly with one of the dancers. When I mentioned it to him, he told me they were 'just really good friends' and, to be honest, I had no reason not to trust him, so I pushed it to the back of my mind.

But it wasn't long before my friend called me again to say Brad had stayed at this girl's house one night, so I challenged him again.

'Oh yeah, I did stay over at her house,' he admitted sheepishly.

'Why?'

'Well, she had a burglary and so she was really scared to stay there on her own, so I offered to stay over.'

'Hmm, I'm not happy about it,' I replied, but I still gave him the benefit of the doubt. I suppose I'd already cottoned on to the fact that he had an eye for the ladies because I'd see him checking out other women when we were out together, so warning signals were starting to go off. Then my friend called again.

'Sorry to tell you this, Bernie, but I saw Bradley with that girl again,' she said.

'What do you mean? What were they doing?'

'Well, they looked really close. They were holding hands and they got into his car together. They looked like a couple.'

That was it. We had a massive row, I told him he was disgusting and that he was a liar and I dumped him.

He kept calling though, so eventually I gave in and agreed to speak to him. He admitted that he'd been wrong to hang out with this girl, but he insisted they were just friends.

'If you're going out with me you can't be walking around Blackpool holding hands with another girl,' I told him. 'I'm very well known there, Bradley, and people love to come and tell me that sort of thing. If you're seeing someone, you just don't do that.'

He fought his corner, so we ended up getting back together and for a while things were fine. I believed him because I wanted to believe him. I was in love.

One night we were together at his house in Abbots Langley and the phone rang, and when he'd finished the call he was crying.

'Jesus, what's happened?' I asked.

'That was her on the phone – that girl from Blackpool – and she's pregnant,' he said tearfully.

I was stunned, but instead of apologising to me or offering some kind of explanation, all he could say was, 'She's all on her own.'

I got up from the sofa, opened the kitchen door and sat on the back step. He followed me outside, but I couldn't bear to look at him. I actually felt sick looking at his face.

'She's on her own is she, Brad? Why's that, then? And what about me, your girlfriend? And what about safe sex?'

I was so shocked, I couldn't even cry.

'There's nothing I can say, is there?' he offered. 'We just got carried away, but I don't want you to leave me. I love you.'

He knew he couldn't worm his way out of this one.

After a sleepless night, I drove back to Blackpool, telling him I needed to be on my own to think things over. He called me every day and he even wrote to me several times to beg my forgiveness and tell me how much he loved me. Eventually, I did forgive him and we got back together.

I knew that an ex-girlfriend sometimes used his house when he was away, which I was OK with because they were never there at the same time. I also decided that as I'd agree to forgive him and move on, I had to learn to trust him again. Our relationship would never work if I was always suspicious about what he was doing.

One day he mentioned his ex had asked to stay at the house one of the weeks he was going to be there.

'Can't you stay somewhere else?' I asked. 'I'm not thrilled about it, Brad – no woman would be.'

His cottage had a quirky layout and you had to walk through the main bedroom to get to the bathroom, so it just wasn't appropriate. However, he told me I was being silly and that he loved me, so I gave in. Again.

A few weeks went by and we were at my house in Loughton in Essex, cleaning up after some tenants had moved out, when Bradley's phone rang. I was in the bedroom when he came in, ashen faced and crying.

'Oh my God, who's died?' I asked panicking. 'Tell me what's happened?'

'That was my ex. She's pregnant.'

I just couldn't believe he'd done it again. We were due to go on holiday to Tenerife the next morning, but instead of calling it off I made him come with me.

'You are coming on holiday and you'll do everything I say.'

On the journey there he was very quiet and very remorseful. I warned him I wasn't going to sleep with him on the holiday, but after about a week and a half I did sleep with him. Looking back, I know I was an idiot and I should have ended the relationship but when you're in love with someone, it's hard to think rationally.

Then, in the summer of 1991, our family was rocked by tragedy when my brother's wife Linzie died suddenly at just twenty-six. She was a dancer, so she was super-fit and didn't drink or smoke. At the time, The Nolans were appearing at the Sandcastle in Blackpool and Linzie had choreographed our show. She popped into our dressing-room on the opening night while I was doing my make-up in front of the mirror. She was standing behind me, so I glanced up at her in the mirror and she just looked like an angel. I'll never forget the feeling I had – she had this amazing glow about her, which almost seemed surreal. She looked absolutely stunning.

'Oh my God, Linzie, you look so beautiful,' I said.

Just a few days later, on the following Monday, Brian called me to say Linzie had a cold.

'Oh no! Give her my love, Brian,' I said, not thinking for one moment it was anything serious. On the Wednesday she still wasn't well, so Brian said he was taking her to the doctor, who gave her Sudafed and sent her home. But when she was lying down she couldn't breathe very well, so on the Thursday Brian took her into hospital and they discovered she had pneumonia. They decided to put her into a coma, so they could drain her lungs.

'Don't worry, Brian,' I said when he called to tell me how she was. 'She's in the right place. They'll look after her and she'll get better.' Then on Friday I got another call from Brian.

'Are you sitting down?' he asked.

'Yes, what's up?'

'Linzie needs a heart transplant.'

The problem wasn't in her lungs. She actually had an undiagnosed heart condition called myocardial infarction. On the Saturday the doctors suggested moving her to a special heart unit at the Victoria Hospital in Manchester, but they warned Brian she might not survive being taken off the life-support machine to make the trip. He had to make the agonising decision of whether or not to risk it, but she needed a heart transplant, so he agreed.

My sisters and I were at Maureen's house in Blackpool, making cups of tea and waiting nervously for an update from the hospital. It was Anne who answered the phone when Brian called to say that Linzie had passed away. It was just six days since she'd started feeling ill with a cold.

It was one of the worst moments of all our lives. It seemed so unfair that this beautiful vibrant girl had been taken away from us. We all loved her like a sister and felt completely devastated. And of course my poor brother was heartbroken. They'd only been married for four years.

The next day I was at Maureen's house when Bradley called. We talked about Linzie for a while and how shocking it was, then he said, 'You know I love you, Bernie, I really do. Will you marry me?'

I was surprised and too upset about Linzie to be excited, but I said yes and added, 'We can't tell anyone for a while, though, because they need time to come to terms with what's happened to Linzie.'

I did love Bradley, but I realise now that our emotions were flying high and what we were feeling wasn't real; it was the result of grief and shock. A tragedy like that makes you reflect on your own life and the people you love, and I think Bradley and I were clinging to each other because we were scared and upset.

A few weeks later I did tell my family and I started to plan a wedding. I got bridal magazines and I even went shopping with my mum and bought a wedding dress. But Bradley just wasn't interested in any of the preparations. I'm sure he'd already started thinking, 'Jesus, what have I done?' We started to row constantly about the wedding. One day I said, 'Come and look at my dress, Brad.'

'I'm not fucking interested in your dress!' he snapped.

'Lovely, but we're supposed to be planning our wedding together.'

It had become obvious that getting married to me wasn't what he wanted, so to save myself any more stress and heartache I suggested we shelved the wedding and luckily the shop took my dress back.

That same summer, I went to Bournemouth for the season with The Nolans, which was a great laugh as we were on the bill alongside Wayne Sleep, Roy Walker and Joe Longthorne. Also in town was a guy called David Ian, who I'd appeared in panto with in Hull a couple of years previously. He was producing a show at the Bournemouth International Centre where we were performing. We'd really hit it off back then and used to go out for a drink after the panto with the rest of the cast. There was never any romance between us, but we both knew we fancied each other. Bradley was in Torquay with his show, so once again we were living in different parts of the country and although our relationship had been limping on, things hadn't been great. So when I bumped into David at the bar in the BIC and he suggested going out the next day, I said, 'Yes, that'd be lovely!'

OK, I was still going out with Bradley but it was rubbish and I thought, 'Screw him, why shouldn't I?' I had no intention of sleeping with David; I just wanted to have a nice day out.

We had a fantastic time – we went for lunch at a gorgeous hotel in Bournemouth, then sat in the bar talking and laughing until about 11 p.m. When I got back to my digs there was a message from Bradley, so I rang him.

'I called you last night, Brad, where were you?' I asked before he had a chance to ask where I'd been all day.

'You won't believe this,' he began. 'But we all went back to this girl's house after the show and I just got too drunk to go home, so I stayed on her couch.'

'Oh, well it's not great really, Brad, considering everything that's happened in the past.'

'I swear to God nothing happened, Bernie. I just slept there and I came home today. We're just good friends.'

At the time Bradley was mates with ex-page-three girl Linda Lusardi, who he'd been in panto with, and her husband. And there was another girl they were friendly with in Bradley's show – a dancer – so the four of them used to go out together for dinner.

I'd already told Bradley I didn't like them going out as a foursome, but he pulled the same old line on me: 'We're just mates, the four of us just get on brilliantly. I'd never go out with her on my own.'

As I'd decided to forgive and forget to give our

relationship a fighting chance, I chose to believe him. What an idiot! The same friend who'd told me about Bradley's shenanigans in Blackpool actually lives in Torquay and told me she'd spotted Bradley in a restaurant with this dancer. 'Oh, yeah, they're friends,' I said, like a fool. 'They go out for dinner with Linda and her husband.'

'Well, Bernie, this was a candlelit restaurant and it was just the two of them at the table.'

'What, do you mean it was just him and her?'

'Well, it looked like a romantic dinner for two to me. I'm just telling you what I saw.'

So I picked up the phone and called Bradley straight away.

'How was your meal last night?' I asked.

'Yeah it was lovely, thanks. The four of us had a great time.'

I knew then he was lying. I took a deep breath before I replied.

'You're lying. There were only two of you there.'

'What the fuck are you talking about?' he snapped.

'You're lying,' I repeated. 'There weren't four of you there.'

'There were! You're mad!'

As usual he'd turned the tables on me, making out that I was crazy.

'You were seen, Bradley, in a candlelit restaurant with that girl. Someone called and told me.'

He had to admit it then. I was supposed to be going down to Torquay to visit him that weekend, so I told him I wouldn't be doing that.

'In fact, Bradley, I don't want to see you any more,' I

said. And I really meant it this time. I felt like a thunder-bolt had hit me and finally made me wake up and realise that he was never going to change – ever. I would never be able to trust him.

'What are you talking about?' he said, clearly gobsmacked. 'I've arranged the whole weekend. Everyone's looking forward to meeting you.'

'Well, I'm not coming. We're over,' I said and hung up.

The truth was, there would always be another woman in Bradley's life somewhere. If he'd decided to get tennis lessons, you could guarantee it would be a woman coaching him! I realised I could never really forgive him for the hurt he'd caused me. I only wish I'd ended our relationship after the first time he cheated – I could have saved myself two or three years of grief. His constant cheating and lying made me feel very insecure about myself for a long time after we broke up. He ended up marrying the dancer he'd been seen with in Torquay, so I guess I wasn't 'mad' after all – there was something going on!

It was a toxic relationship in lots of ways. It was very fiery and sometimes even bordered on violent, which could be scary. He had a bad temper and so did I. Physically, he was a very passionate person – which was great when we were getting along, and the sexual side of our relation-ship was probably what kept pulling us back together, but it could also be destructive.

He was genuinely shocked that I'd dumped him and wrote to me in Bournemouth saying how devastated he was that I could think he was up to something with that dancer. He said I was the love of his life and that he hoped we could be friends. I wrote back to him saying, 'I don't want to be your friend, Bradley. I wanted to be your wife. I've got loads of friends.'

I knew the only way to move on was for me to have nothing to do with him – I'd learnt that tip from Bob. I think it helped that I'd bumped into David Ian again because he made me realise I could have feelings for someone else. I had very strong feelings for David and we ended up seeing each other on and off for about a year, but he was always so busy as he'd just started his own theatre production company – which is now huge – and I was touring so much we hardly saw each other. I think David also worried I'd end up back with Bradley and that he'd get hurt. I was upset when we split up, but it was for the best and we've remained good friends.

After David, I dated a friend of Shane's called Mickey Salmon for a few months. He was a comedian and a really lovely guy, but it was never right between us, so we didn't last long. I think I was on the rebound. Tragically, Mickey died suddenly about a year after we broke up – it turned out he had a condition similar to that of my sister-in-law Linzie. Apparently, he collapsed as he was going through the turnstiles at an Arsenal match.

In 1993 The Nolans were doing a summer season in Weymouth and I was single again. When I'd been with Bradley we could never get work together, so we always ended up in different resorts for the summer season. But this year suddenly he was on the same bill! I couldn't believe it. And, perhaps inevitably, during the first week of the show I ended up sleeping with him and we very nearly got back together. There had always been a big sexual pull between us, I suppose, and we had really loved each other. But while I didn't have anyone to answer to, Bradley had a girlfriend. Of course he kept promising he was going to finish with her, but three weeks later he still hadn't told her.

In the meantime, someone else had caught my eye – Steve Doneathy, who was the drummer in our band. I'd first met Steve in 1991 when The Nolans played Butlins in Ayr and our regular drummer couldn't make it, so the keyboard player suggested Steve. We all had our little job in the group – Maureen was in charge of clothes, Anne was in charge of money and I was in charge of music and the band, while Coleen got away with doing nothing! She loved that. So I agreed to Steve playing with us, but on the day of our first soundcheck he was two hours late. He'd never played with us before so I was worried about the gig – and angry! It turned out there was some problem with the traffic, but when Steve eventually got there we talked through the music with our MD and then he started playing and didn't put a foot wrong – he was absolutely brilliant. I was very impressed

We never got to know each other that well, though. Sometimes we'd go out with the band and have a meal before the show and I always thought Steve was a really good guy, but I never thought of him as a potential boyfriend. Plus he was going out with someone else at the time. But I think he must have fancied me a bit because when we played G-A-Y in 1992 and I was with Mickey Salmon, Steve saw him coming into the dressingroom and told me later he thought to himself, 'How the hell did he pull her?'

Then in Weymouth we started getting to know each other better. Every night after the show we'd all pile into the bar and stay there until four or five in the morning! There were four of us who were considered the life and soul of the party – the comedian Johnny Casson, Bradley, Steve and me. As long as one of us was there everyone was happy. Steve was quite a flirt actually. I used to catch him staring at me from across the bar and because he was so funny and could always make me laugh, I began to really like him. He was handsome too – tall and dark.

One day Bradley came over to me and told me his girl-friend had turned up unexpectedly. 'Bradley, she's your girlfriend, she's entitled to turn up,' I said.

'She's only going to be here this weekend and I'm going to tell her about us,' he promised.

Well, she was there for a month and during that time I decided I wasn't going to be messed about by him again. I was much stronger at that point and I'd been getting closer to Steve. He used to walk me home because my digs were right next to the house he was renting. It was so romantic, walking along the river and across the bridge, and one night, when we'd stopped to look at the boats, he turned to me. 'Can I kiss you?' he asked.

'Don't ask, just do it!' I said. He walked me to my door every night from then on and eventually he stayed over and we got together.

I realised straight away that Steve had a load of good qualities – he was strong and independent, but loyal and reliable too.

Bradley found out that Steve and I had started seeing

each other and one night he said to Coleen backstage, 'Tell your sister she's a lunatic.'

'I think you'll find you are the lunatic, Bradley,' she told him. 'You were supposed to finish with your girlfriend a month ago. What do you expect?'

I like to think that what happened between Bradley and me made him realise he was in love with his girlfriend, and I was happy that I'd got together with Steve, so things worked out for the best.

After that season in Weymouth, Steve was booked to work on a cruise ship. We had a last night party and the next morning we had to say goodbye and go our separate ways. As I watched him drive off, I felt really desolate. I already felt something deep – for me it hadn't been just a casual fling – and I knew I was really going to miss him.

He wrote to me nearly every day from the ship and called when he could, too. When he came home I was back living with my friend Dee in Blackpool, so we spent some time there and it was lovely to be together again. But for the first year of our relationship Steve was working on the ship on and off, which meant we were apart quite a lot. It was great when I got to visit him on board as his guest, although his quarters were bloody awful! His cabin was way down in the depths of the ship, so if there was any bad weather you could really feel it and we'd frequently get thrown out of bed! We'd snuggle into the bunk and lie there while the ship was rolling round, laughing and trying not to throw up.

We had so much fun. I used to watch his show every night and I met a fantastic comedian called Tommy Sutton and another couple called Emily and Phil Bell – she was a singer on the cruise and her husband played drums. Steve and I had been getting really close and I'd booked to cruise with him to Venice. My friend Drew said to me one day, 'Do you think Steve will propose to you on the Venice cruise? And if he does, what will you say?'

'I have no idea if he'll propose, but I'd say yes,' I replied. Steve was different to the other guys I'd been out with. Our relationship was passionate and exciting, but there was also trust, loyalty and respect. I knew he cared about me deeply and would never hurt me. I was head over heels in love with him.

'Oh my God! He will! I know he's going to propose to you!' said Drew, who was almost as excited as I was about the idea!

The day I was flying out to Venice to see Steve, I had an audition for a stage production of *Billy Liar* with my friend David Ian's company. We had to do a comedy piece, so I put together a few sketches from Victoria Wood's books which, without wishing to sound bigheaded, were really bloody good! I explained to David that I had to catch a flight and begged him not to run late. After my audition, they asked me to hang around. 'Oh God, typical!' I thought. Usually it would be great news to be asked to stay behind, but all I could think about was catching my flight to see Steve. My friend Drew was also at the auditions, as he was up for the part of Arthur, so we waited nervously together.

'God Drew, I'm going to miss my flight!' I kept saying, checking my watch every five seconds. And then David came back into the room.

'Don't worry,' he said. 'We're going to get you back in first because I've told them you need to catch a plane.'

As always, David couldn't have been lovelier. I had to go back and do more singing and acting, but almost before they'd had a chance to say, 'Thanks Bernie, we'll be in touch,' I was halfway out the door and on my way to the airport. Just as I arrived, my agent called to say I'd got the part of Rita in *Billy Liar*, so when I boarded the plane that day I was buzzing with excitement. 'If Steve asks me to marry him now, my life will be perfect,' I thought.

Before the trip I'd bought this gorgeous suit with a tight pencil skirt and I was wearing it when Steve met me at the airport. He told me later when he saw me walking towards him that day he couldn't get over how gorgeous I looked; it was the moment he realised he didn't want anyone else to have me.

But he didn't ask me to marry him! We had a fantastic time in Venice though, and when I got home I decided that if he didn't pop the question on the next cruise, then I was going to ask him to marry me!

On the next cruise the ship was docking at Venice again for a day, so Steve suggested we went out to dinner. This time I had my own beautiful cabin – Tommy Sutton and his wife Jo were also on the ship and they each had a cabin, so Jo gave me hers and Steve put a huge bouquet of flowers and a beautiful bottle of wine in there. It was very romantic.

That night I got dressed up, and as we were leaving I noticed everyone was grinning and saying, 'See ya! Have a good meal!' I remember thinking, 'That's weird they're taking such an interest.' It didn't actually cross my mind that Steve was planning something.

We walked around the streets of Venice for ages, trying to find the restaurant, then when we finally came across it and sat down to eat, the service was unbelievably slow. I saw Steve was getting really worked up, but the ship wasn't leaving till midnight, so we had plenty of time – or so I thought!

'Steve, stop getting so agitated, you're going to ruin the night,' I said. 'What's the matter? Calm down.'

'They're taking too long, it's ridiculous, we've got to get back on the ship at twelve.'

'Yeah and it's half past seven, half an hour since the last time you looked at the time!' I said.

When our food finally arrived, Steve rushed me through it and before I knew it he'd paid the bill and he was ushering me out the door.

'I want to take you somewhere special. Come on, follow me,' he said, taking my hand.

He was looking for the Rialto Bridge, but couldn't find it. Once you get lost in Venice, you get really lost because the little narrow streets all look the same. By this time it was about 10.30 p.m. and it would take a bit of time to get back to the ship.

'Look Steve, don't worry about the Rialto,' I said.

'I want to find it!' he insisted. It was like a comedy sketch, as he dragged me around while I did my best not to topple over in my heels. Eventually, we got to a pretty little square and Steve stopped and turned towards me.

'I can't find the Rialto Bridge, but . . . do you love me?' he said.

'Of course I do! I'm a bit out of breath and I'm slightly annoyed with you for rushing through dinner then dragging me around the streets of Venice, but I do love you.'

'I don't suppose you'd consider spending the rest of your life with me, would you?'

'What?'

'Will you marry me?'

'Yes!' I was so thrilled.

We didn't have much time to enjoy the moment, though, because we had to get back to the ship. We needed to find a taxi boat fast, so Steve grabbed my hand and we started running again! It turned out it was going to cost us £100 to get back to the port and we only had £50 in cash on us.

'We're going to miss the ship and we've just got engaged,' pleaded Steve.

'Get in,' said the taxi driver, starting the engine, and we sped off to the dock under a blanket of stars, hugging and kissing at the back of the boat.

When we got there they were just about to pull the last gangplank up. Our friends were all sitting at the back of the ship with champagne on ice ready for our return. 'Well?' asked Tommy and Jo when they saw us.

'She said yes!' said Steve with a big grin on his face. Everyone knew what he'd been planning. We cracked open the bubbly and had a toast. It was a great moment because even though it wasn't planned, the speedboat trip back to the dock made it so exciting and special.

The ship was going on to Rhodes that night, so we decided to shop for my engagement ring there. The whole trip was just fabulous. The only downer was finding out that *Billy Liar* had been cancelled when I got home. I was devastated about it, but at least I got severance pay.

Apart from getting engaged, a couple of other big things happened in 1994. It was the year I bought my house in Blackpool – a gorgeous little semi-detached, which meant Steve and I had our own place to retreat to. I also left The Nolans. Coleen had left the year before to be a mum and, to be honest, I hadn't been enjoying it for a while. All the cabaret clubs had closed down and we weren't big enough to do proper tours – it had been a long time since we'd had a hit record. After Coleen left we started slogging around discos and bingo halls and we made hardly any money. We'd got rid of our lighting and crew. Eventually we got rid of the band and started using backing tapes and that was the final straw for me. We did a summer season with The Grumbleweeds at the Grand in Blackpool and that's when I told the other girls I'd had enough.

'I'm going to leave after this season. I can't do it any more,' I admitted. 'I'm not doing the sort of gigs I want to do any more.'

I felt terrible because I was leaving Anne and Maureen on their own, but it was the right decision for me. I had to try to build my own career away from the group.

The first couple of years after leaving were really tough, though. Being a Nolan sister was a disadvantage rather than an advantage and I really struggled to get work. But I was happy with Steve and he was happy to pay the mortgage while I kept trying to get a break. That's what being a couple is all about – working as a team to support each other.

We set a date to get married – 25 May 1996. I wanted the proper big white wedding. I didn't go for a Catholic service; I went for a Church of England church in Blackpool because it had the best grounds!

The night before the wedding I stayed at my house with my sister Coleen, who was my chief bridesmaid, and the next morning the rest of the girls came round to get ready. Then we all got taxis round to my parents' house in Waterloo Road where I'd grown up and Dad made us bacon and eggs. 'You've got to have a full breakfast!' he insisted. And we washed it down with Buck's Fizz! Dad wasn't very well that day, though, and I remember thinking he looked a bit poorly.

All the neighbours were out in the street waiting for us to come out. My mum and sisters left first, so I was left with Dad on my own for a few moments.

'So are you happy and do you love him?' he asked.

'Oh yeah, I'm so happy, Dad.'

'Then I'm happy for you. You've always been a great daughter and I hope you have a wonderful life together.' It was a special moment between my dad and me.

When we got to the church, all of Steve's immediate family were late apart from his brother Robert. I was so calm, though, that when he suggested we just went ahead without them, I laughed.

'Robert, calm down. We're not going to do anything without your family. We'll just wait.'

Luckily it wasn't raining, and eventually they arrived and rushed past us into the church.

The service was lovely. My mum sang 'A Prayer Perfect' beautifully and my sisters and brothers sang 'One Hand,

One Heart' from *West Side Story* and 'You My Love' *a capella*. Everyone in the church was crying!

The reception was at the Grand Hotel in St Anne's. We had a live band and we sang, danced and drank until four in the morning. At one point I was sitting on top of the piano in the hotel lobby in my wedding dress, belting out a tune at the top of my voice.

'Um, Mrs Doneathy,' ventured the manager nervously. 'I'm going to have to ask you to go to bed now because my other guests are complaining.'

It was marvellous! We couldn't go on honeymoon because Steve was working on *Summer Holiday* in Blackpool at the time, so the next day everyone came round to my house and we had another big shindig, which sadly Steve had to miss to go to work.

I loved being married right from day one and I still love it. I believe in marriage as an institution and think it's a wonderful thing to find a partner for life. And I did feel different once I had that ring on my finger – I felt even closer to Steve.

The following summer, I finally got a job! I landed a role in *Oh What a Night* in Blackpool and I also got asked to do my own cabaret show at the Sutcliffe Hotel in Blackpool. So after appearing in *Oh What a Night*, I used to get straight into a taxi to do the cabaret. It was hard work, but I loved being back on stage and it enabled Steve and me to buy a bigger house on Charlotte Avenue in St Anne's. We loved our new home – it was beautiful with big bright rooms and a huge garden. Things were looking up.

5

MY DAUGHTERS

....

I was never one of those girls who longed for babies. I knew I wanted kids one day, but they weren't the be all and end all. However, when Steve announced that he didn't want children the year before we got married, I realised I didn't want to fall in love with someone who didn't want a family. It was such a big issue that we actually split up over it, but Steve called me after a few days apart and said, 'Look, with you I do want to have kids.'

I was thirty-seven when we started trying for a baby and, being that bit older, I wasn't sure how easy it was going to be to conceive or if I'd be able to get pregnant at all, so I knew I had to get on with it. I bought an ovulation kit from the chemist to pinpoint my most fertile days and took it with us when we went on holiday to the South of France with Maureen and Ritchie.

Well, it did the trick, because when I got back home, I found out I was pregnant and Steve and I couldn't have been more delighted.

We decided to wait until Christmas time when the family

was all gathered at the house in Waterloo Road to share our good news.

'We've got something to tell you . . . I'm pregnant!'

Everyone started screaming and throwing their arms round Steve and me, and my dad pretended to faint! They were all so excited, which was lovely for us.

For a while, everything was going along fine with the pregnancy. I didn't suffer from morning sickness and we were enjoying living in our lovely house in St Anne's. I was reading baby books and planning how we'd decorate the nursery – it was a really exciting time.

I'd also recently landed the role of Mrs Johnstone in a touring production of *Blood Brothers*, but I felt good and had loads of energy, and the cast and crew looked after me really well.

In May 1998 I went to the Victoria Hospital in Blackpool for a routine twenty-week scan. As she was scanning me, the sonographer kept frowning.

'I can't see the baby properly because of the position it's in. Can you have a walk around and come back?'

So Steve and I went outside and walked around for five minutes. When I got back on the bed for another scan, the sonographer still looked confused as she stared at the monitor.

'I'll have to go and get one of my colleagues to come and speak to you,' she said and left the room.

She came back with a doctor a few minutes later.

'We're not happy with the scan, I'm afraid,' said the doctor.

'What does that mean?' I asked, feeling sick.

'Well, your baby isn't developing properly. It's very small

for twenty weeks, so I'd like you to have an amniocentesis in Manchester today.'

Steve and I drove to St Mary's Hospital in Manchester, stunned by what had happened. I had more scans and the amniocentesis, which is where they put a needle through your belly button and take a sample of amniotic fluid. After the tests, I got dressed and Steve and I waited for the doctor.

She finally emerged, carrying a stack of scans. 'I hate to tell you this, but I think your baby might have Down's syndrome,' she said gently. 'We won't know for sure until we get the results of the amniocentesis, which will be in about a week's time.'

Steve and I were so shocked we could hardly speak as the doctor showed us the scans and explained the baby wasn't developing normally and had a hole in its heart, too.

When we got home to St Anne's, all we could think about was what we'd do if our baby did have Down's syndrome. Would we have the baby? Did we have the strength and the skills to look after a child with such great needs? It was dreadful.

In the end, the decision was taken out of our hands. A week later, the doctor from the Victoria Hospital called us at home.

'We've got the results of the tests and it's not Down's syndrome,' she said.

At first my heart leapt because I thought it was good news, but she quickly dashed my hopes.

'It's actually worse, I'm afraid. Your baby has a very rare condition called Edward's syndrome. It's a chromosome disorder that results in very serious disabilities.'

The list was endless – hole in the heart, cleft palate, club foot, spina bifida, no neck, severe learning disabilities. When I put the phone down, Steve and I looked out on to our garden and I just collapsed in his arms and cried. I sobbed my heart out – we both did. We were heartbroken.

Not long afterwards my friend Frank Wilcox called me. At the time, he was a consultant obstetrician at the Victoria Hospital.

'Children with Edward's syndrome don't survive, Bernie,' he said gently.

'What do you mean?'

'Even if you go ahead with the pregnancy and have this baby, it will die. There is never any other scenario. Very few survive for more than a year and most only live a few hours or days after the birth. Obviously you can say no, but I can book you in to be induced tomorrow.'

I trusted Frank – he was a close friend, as well as an expert in his field.

'Is that what you would do, Frank?' I asked.

'Personally, I think it's best for all of you. If you go the full nine months, you will feel your baby kicking inside you and you will have grown more attached to it. You might have the child for a week and it will be in pain and then it will die.'

I just couldn't bear the thought of my baby suffering, so I agreed to have the labour induced the next day at the Victoria Hospital. I was five and a half months pregnant.

The next day, Steve and I made a very sombre journey to the hospital. Once there, we were shown into a special

SANDS room for the labour. SANDS is the Stillbirth and Neonatal Death Society charity. The room was lovely, with an en suite and a sofa bed so that Steve could stay with me. It was right next to the maternity unit though, so I could hear women giving birth and babies crying, and laughter.

Steve and me had dinner together that night in the room. I'd been given medication to induce the birth, and later that evening I went into labour.

I'll never forget one thing the nurse said, and I know she didn't mean to upset me, but it stuck in my mind and I wanted to hit her. She came in to check on me and said, 'The baby's just sitting there.'

Obviously the baby was already dead, but it felt like such an insensitive thing to say at the time.

'You can push now,' said the nurse, so I pushed a few times, and with one huge push my baby was delivered. The worst thing of all was that the room was silent, except for the sound of Steve quietly sobbing.

'Would you like to know the sex?' asked the nurse.

'Yes please.'

'It's a girl. I'll take her away to wash her, but would you like me to bring her back so you can see her?'

'Yes.' I wanted to see my baby.

When the nurse came back the baby was in a tiny basket and wrapped in a little blanket with a white hat on her head. 'She's ready for you to see,' she said.

'Can you tell me what she looks like, so I'm prepared?' I asked. I knew she wasn't fully developed and I was worried I'd be upset by what I saw.

'Well, she's very, very pink and very tiny, and one of

her eyes is open. It's up to you whether you see her, but I think she looks very cute.'

I wasn't allowed to touch her or pick her up because she was too fragile, but when the nurse pulled the blanket back I could see she had long legs and long fingers like her dad.

Steve and I decided to call her Kate. I'd always loved Katherine Hepburn and we both thought Kate was a lovely name.

'Would you like to have her baptised?' asked the nurse.

Steve and I aren't religious people, but at that stage I did believe in God so I said yes and told her I'd been brought up Catholic.

'Well, I can tell you now, no one from the Catholic Church will come because they'll consider it an abortion,' she explained gently.

To be honest, that's when I really lost all faith. If that's what it meant to be Catholic, then it wasn't for me.

The nurse arranged for a female reverend from the Church of England to come and baptise Kate later that day, and she said some beautiful words for our little girl. Steve was utterly devastated and sobbed uncontrollably in my arms. I didn't cry then, and I'm not really sure why that was. But I felt it was important to be strong for Steve and to comfort him because men often get forgotten in these situations.

We got to spend about five hours with Kate and we took some pictures to remember her by. I've got a special box at home that contains her photographs and all the cards that were sent to us when she died. We had a funeral for Kate, but only Steve and me went and the lovely

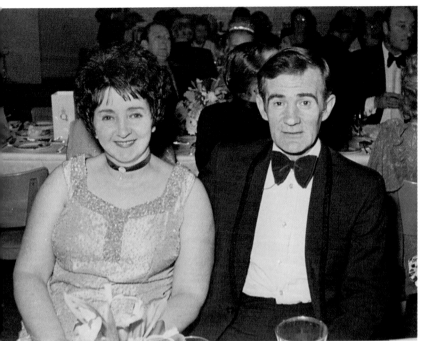

My parents – Maureen and Tommy Nolan. Despite their ups
and downs they were together for over fifty years.

Me aged 4 years old. I had already been
singing and performing for two years!

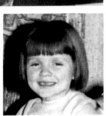

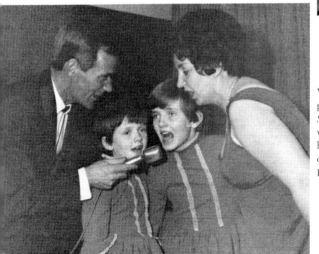

When we first
performed as *The
Singing Nolans*
we would sing
harmonies together
on show songs.
I loved it!

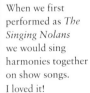

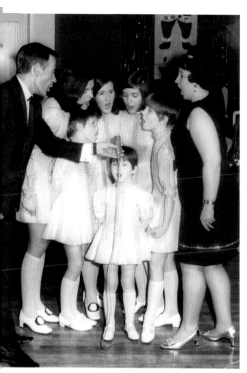

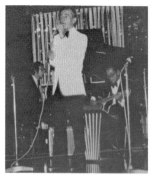

My father loved to sing Frank Sinatra songs at our shows.

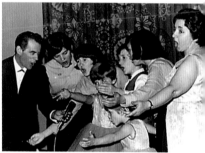

Here we are all singing together. Clockwise from top left we are Dad, Anne, Denise, Maureen, Linda, Mum, Coleen and me.

Our early gigs were at posh London hotels like the Grosvenor House Hotel, or at Labour clubs around the country.

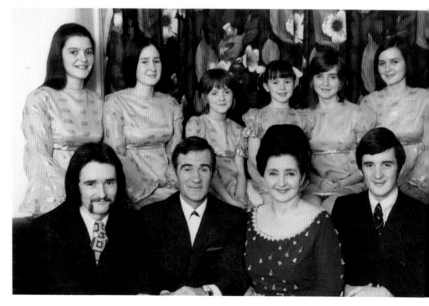

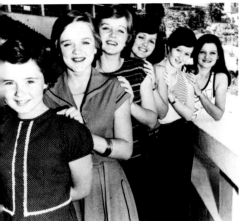

Linda and I were always close because we were so near in age, with only 20 months between us. We both looked out for Coleen (in the middle here), as she was the baby of the family. This was taken at our school in Ilford, Essex.

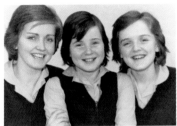

We became *The Nolan Sisters* and moved to London in 1974, when I was just thirteen years old.

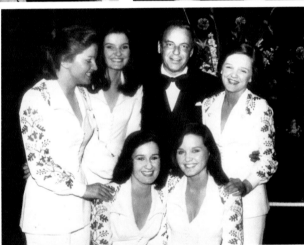

Going on tour with Frank Sinatra was an incredible experience. Here we are with Frank in 1975.

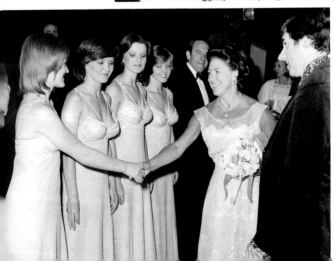

Meeting Princess Margaret after a show.

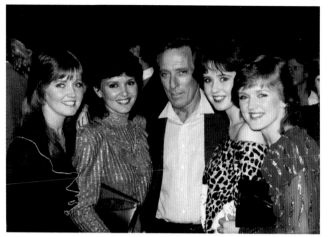

We were lucky enough to work with some amazing people. Here are my sisters and I with Andy Williams, whom we often performed with. This was taken in Japan in 1980.

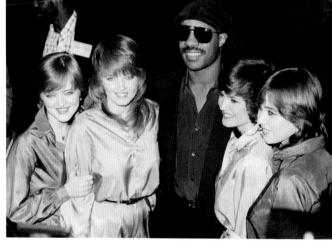

Here we are with Stevie Wonder, just after we had won the Tokyo Music Festival Competition in 1981.

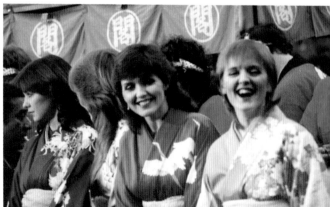

On tour in Japan that same year.

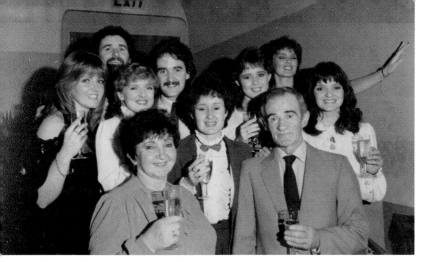

he whole family celebrating together. We had a
reat time whenever we went on tour.

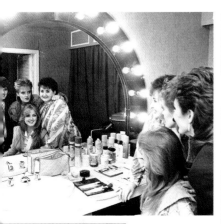

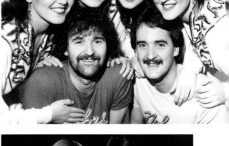

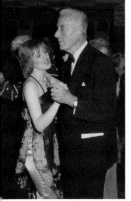

Dancing with Lord
Mountbatten.

Here we are
appearing on
the Devon
News Service,
with Anne's
daughter Amy.

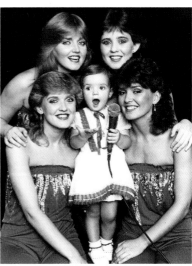

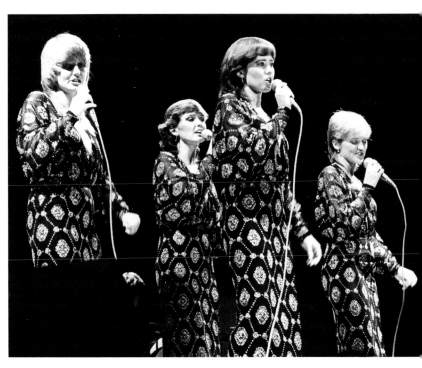

At first I hated our matching outfits – but I grew to love them!

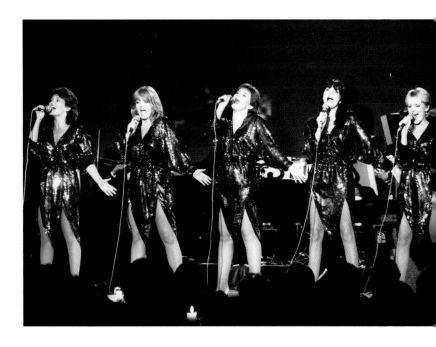

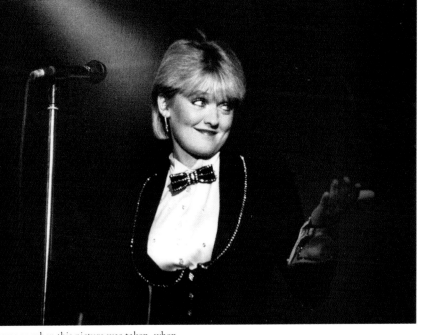

was 22 when this picture was taken, when
we were on tour in the UK in 1982.

Me and my old boyfriend Bob on holiday in
Hawaii. It didn't work out between us but he
was very loyal, kind and funny.

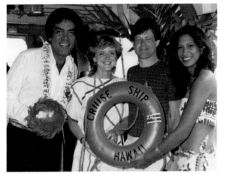

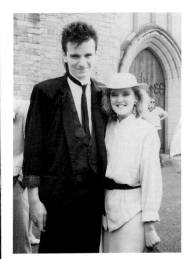

Here I am with Gavin at my brother's
wedding. Gavin had dated Coleen
before me, so it was a little awkward
when we got together!

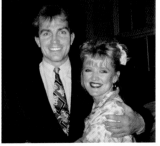

Me and Brad in Blackpool in
1991. We had a very tempestuous
relationship.

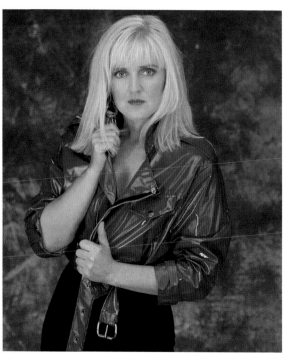

Looking glamorous in the eighties!

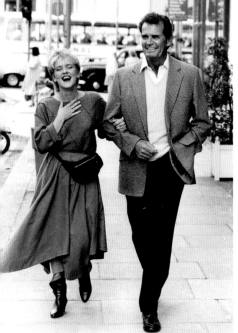

I met the American actor James Garner filming the *Bob Hope Classic* live TV show.

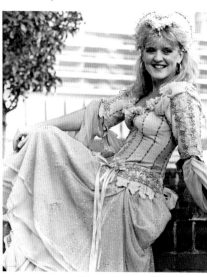

I have always loved doing panto. Here I am dressed as Maid Marion in *Babes in the Wood* at the Birmingham Hippodrome in 1989.

reverend who'd baptised her. She was buried in the same churchyard in Blackpool where my sister-in-law Linzie was buried. The funeral directors handed Steve Kate's tiny white coffin and he carried it to the graveside, which was really, really sad to see. The reverend said some nice words and we placed flowers on the grave. I kept one of the flowers, which I pressed and put in the box alongside Kate's other things.

After the funeral, we went back to our house in St Anne's and I invited my close family over for some food. It was a beautiful sunny day in May, so we sat in the back garden. I'd put all Kate's flowers and a few photographs of her in one of the bedrooms upstairs, and Anne, Denise and Maureen asked if they could go up and see her.

'Yes, it's fine, but I have to warn you, she's very pink and her eye is open, but she has lovely little hands and long legs.'

So they went upstairs and looked at Kate's picture, and they all cried. I remember my dad knocked on the bedroom door and when I opened it he said, 'I've put a blazer on. Am I alright to come in?' As if I wouldn't let him in because he wasn't dressed right!

It was actually a lovely day. It was sad of course, but it was nice to have my family around me and I really felt I'd done the best thing for Kate.

After everyone had gone that day, Steve and I had a little cry. We were exhausted. We went to bed early that night and said a little prayer for Kate, then fell asleep in each other's arms.

* * *

I felt very down after Kate's death, but as far as I could see there were only two choices – carry on with life or kill myself, and killing myself just wasn't an option. Life is precious and I owed it to Kate to move on. I never wanted counselling – I could always talk to my sisters and we'd said our goodbyes to Kate in a way that felt right for us. She would never be forgotten, but I didn't want to constantly go over what had happened – I think dwelling on things in that way would have made me feel worse.

My way of healing and moving on was to go back on tour with *Blood Brothers*, which I did a week after I buried Kate. Steve and I had been sitting around at home, staring at the four walls like two zombies. I knew we had to snap out of it somehow, so I decided to go back to work and Steve came with me. It was very cathartic actually, because in the play two children die and from then on those tears I shed on stage were real. I could express how I felt every night and I didn't need any help with crying on cue. My sisters came to see me in it and they knew they were real tears, so they were sobbing too.

Kate's death brought Steve and me closer both emotionally and physically. We had this powerful need to be close and give each other as much love as we could, in every way we knew how, and by July I was pregnant again. I was so happy, but nervous that something might be wrong with this pregnancy too.

I was also worried about my dad. He had a lung disease similar to emphysema and had to carry an oxygen tank around with him. He was a very proud man, though, so you'd hardly ever see him with it. I wanted him to come and see me in *Blood Brothers*, but he wouldn't come with his oxygen tank.

He began to get more and more out of breath and eventually he was sitting on the steps at home with Mum and he couldn't breathe at all, so she called an ambulance. My dad never came out of hospital. It was September and I was on tour with *Blood Brothers* in Glasgow when I got a phone call to say he'd been taken into hospital. Because it was the opening night of a new tour, we didn't have any understudies so I went on stage that night and told my family to keep me posted.

It was Maureen who called to tell me Dad had passed away. Fortunately, I'd gone back to Blackpool and seen him about a week before he died and we'd chatted and had a hug. I was glad that he knew I was pregnant again and he'd been delighted for Steve and me. He died on a Wednesday morning and I performed in the matinee that afternoon because they didn't have an understudy and they would have had to cancel the show. My dad wouldn't have wanted that, so I went on stage and travelled back that night after the show. When I got home to Blackpool, I got a phone call from Bill Kenwright's office, the production company behind *Blood Brothers*, telling me that if I wasn't back at work on Friday I'd get the sack.

'Listen to me,' I said to the woman on the other end of the phone, trying to contain my anger. 'I'll come back to work on Monday after my dad gets buried. That's it; there are no ifs or buts. If you don't want me back, I won't come back,' then I hung up.

It made that weekend even harder for me because not only had I just lost my dad, but I thought I'd lost my job as well. When I spoke to Bill Kenwright about it after-wards, he told me he had no idea that's what I'd been told. I love my job with a passion, but the business can be horrible. There are some notable exceptions to the rule, but generally show business is full of people who'll stab you in the back as quick as look at you. Tony Clayman, who was my agent for twenty-one years and a lovely man, always told me the most important thing I could do was to hang on to my integrity and keep my feet on the ground, and I'd like to think that I've been able to do that.

It was terrible after Dad died. There's no doubt he had many faults, but he was also the lynchpin of our family, whether we liked it or not. We used to go to him with good news and talk to him about the shows and gigs we'd done. I knew he loved us and we loved him.

My mum in particular was never the same after Dad died and I'm convinced the shock and grief over his death brought on her Alzheimer's, although it took a while to become apparent. She missed him so much, even though they'd argued all the time and in their youth he'd messed around with other women and, of course, been violent towards her. But his death left a massive hole in her life because, no matter what else went on, they'd done every-thing together. At the end Dad kept saying how much he loved Mum, but he didn't realise it until it was too late.

At my three-month scan, the doctors weren't happy with what they saw. It felt like history was repeating itself and it looked like my worst fears were about to be realised. They weren't sure exactly what was wrong, though. I had an amniocentesis, but the results were inconclusive. They speculated the baby could have Prader-Willi syndrome, which causes restricted growth and learning disabilities or something else called floppy baby syndrome, but they would need to do another amniocentesis to be sure. I remember thinking, 'What the hell is wrong with us?'

I had the test again and then went back on tour with *Blood Brothers*, which was in Nottingham that week. Work was the only thing keeping me sane.

On the day the hospital was going to call with the results, Steve and I were walking around a shop called the Pier, trying to distract ourselves, when my mobile rang. It was a nurse from the hospital so I went outside to take the call.

'I've got your results Mrs Doneathy,' she said.

'OK, tell me what they are,' I replied, bracing myself for bad news.

'There was a fault with the first amniocentesis they did. Your baby is absolutely normal.'

I immediately cried with joy and relief. I phoned my mum and my brothers and sisters to tell them the good news and they were all delighted for us. After that, my pregnancy went smoothly and I even managed to avoid morning sickness.

I had planned to have a natural water birth with my favourite music playing in the background, but in the end my obstetrician Frank Wilcox decided to induce me because I was two days overdue and he didn't want to take any risks after what happened with Kate. So I went into hospital and was given a pessary to induce the labour at about 10 p.m., then around midnight I started getting contractions.

'Arrgh! Steve, I think I'm in labour,' I said through gritted teeth.

'Don't be silly, it's only been two hours since the pessary.'

'I'm telling you, this is labour!'

When the nurse examined me I was in labour, so I was wheeled down to the delivery room. 'Er, where's the birthing pool?' I asked.

'Oh no, you can't go in the pool if you've been induced.'

So much for my birth plan!

I ended up being in labour for ten hours with just gas and air to take the edge off the pain. But eventually, I said, 'Right, I can't bear this any more. I need you to do something now Steve!'

'What can I do?' he said.

The baby's heartbeat started dropping, so my friend Frank Wilcox said, 'Here's the situation: you can have an epidural and I'll take you down now for a caesarean, and Steve can get into scrubs and come in. But if you don't make a decision now, I'll pull you out, you'll have the C-section under a general anaesthetic and Steve won't be there.'

I looked at Steve and he just looked back at me with wide eyes and his gob open. 'Just do it, just take me down now,' I said, laughing. I think the gas and air was working!

The caesarean was over so quickly and I didn't feel a thing.

'It's a girl!' said Frank, holding the baby up so I could see her.

'Oh my God, she's so like Steve, it's scary!' I said.

She was born on 26 April 1999, weighing 8lbs 7oz and had a shock of black hair like Steve (although he's since gone bald!). She was the spit of him. I've never seen a child more like their father – ever! And she still is, although her hair is now blonde.

The nurse put her on to my breast to start feeding, and I'll never forget that feeling of pure love and happiness as I held my gorgeous little girl. It was amazing; Steve and I both felt so lucky to have her. We decided to call her Erin and gave her Kate as a middle name in memory of her sister.

It felt wonderful taking her home to our house in St Anne's where we'd decorated her nursery in a Winnie the Pooh theme. I took to motherhood pretty well. In fact, just a week after the caesarean Steve's mum came to visit us and we went out shopping with Erin in her new pram. I was so proud and happy.

She was a really good baby, but breastfeeding was a nightmare at first. I had scabs for a month and bled every time she latched on. It was so painful I cried my eyes out! Steve begged me to use a bottle, but I was determined to persevere. In the end I breastfed Erin for seven months.

I went back on tour with *Blood Brothers* just three months after giving birth and Steve and Erin came with me. We managed to make it work and became a really tight little unit. I finally had my own family and I was doing a job I loved. Life doesn't get any better than that.

6
FROM *BROOKSIDE* TO *THE BILL*

....

At the beginning of 2000 I got a call from my agent Tony to tell me that the producer of the Channel 4 soap *Brookside*, Paul Marquess, wanted me to audition for a part on the show.

'Really?' I asked, wondering why on earth he'd picked me, because apart from a bit of rep theatre, I'd always done musicals. Singing had always been my thing and I wasn't known as a straight actress.

Tony went on to explain that a new family was being introduced – the Murrays – and they were looking for someone to play the mother, Diane.

'OK, well I'll go for the audition,' I told Tony. 'But I'm pretty sure I won't get it.'

It turned out that Paul had seen me in *Blood Brothers* at Christmas, when the show was in Liverpool. Bill Kenwright usually replaced the girl who played Mrs Johnstone on the tour with the West End Mrs J for Liverpool, which is the show's home city. But that year he said he wanted me to play the part, which I was really chuffed about. The show's creator, Willy Russell, came along and he told me I was in his top two Mrs J's – what a privilege! And Paul was there with some other execs from *Brookside*, who all thought I'd be a brilliant Diane. They loved my Scouse accent!

So I went along for the audition, which was a bit scary because it was all on camera. I had to film a scene with four different guys who were up for the part of Marty Murray, Diane's husband. In the scene, we got the keys to our new house on the Close and Marty has to pick up Diane and whirl her around, shouting, 'We've got the keys!' One of the guys was an actor called Neil Caple, who was a total natural.

When I got back to the theatre for the matinee, my phone rang and it was Tony to tell me that *Brookside* had offered me a three-year contract.

'Oh my God!' I really hadn't expected to get the part. 'But I've just signed up to do *Blood Brothers* for a year in the West End. How's that going to work?'

'Well, Bernie, I think I should try to get you out of that contract because this is TV and it's a big show,' said Tony.

When I came off the phone, I sat in my dressingroom trying to work out how I felt about a part with no singing. I realised that I actually felt excited about doing something different.

But when it came to getting out of my contract, Bill was having none of it and told Tony he'd sue me. I decided to write to Bill myself.

'Dear Bill, I'm writing to the part of you that was once a performer and entertainer,' I began. 'I really feel this is a great opportunity for me. I know *Blood Brothers* is fantastic and I've learned so much from it, but this is an opportunity to do something that goes out to millions of people and I'd really like to try it.'

Bill wrote back, saying he thought I was mad for wanting to leave *Blood Brothers*, but he agreed to let me go and even told me there would always be a place for me on the show. It was very good of him.

Steve and I were in the process of buying a gorgeous six-bedroom house near Lytham in Lancashire, so getting the *Brookside* job meant I would be able to commute to Liverpool every day. It was perfect.

My first day on set involved a full on-screen kiss with my 'husband' Marty (aka Neil Caple, who'd got the part). I hadn't kissed another man since I'd got together with Steve – on or off screen!

I was in my dressingroom, thinking, 'Right, I'm not Bernie Nolan, I am Diane Murray . . . I am Diane Murray. If you want them to believe you, make it believable. Believe it yourself.'

Little did I know that Neil was in another room, thinking, 'She's not one of the Nolans, she's Diane Murray. She's not one of the Nolans, she's Diane Murray!' We only realised what we'd both been thinking when we talked about it afterwards.

We did the kiss and it was completely fine. Neil is such a great actor and I ended up learning so much from him during my time on the show. The Murrays had some meaty storylines which I could get stuck into, including their attempts to have a baby through fertility treatment.

A couple of months after joining *Brookside*, I had a miscarriage at work when I was around ten weeks pregnant. I was on set when I suddenly felt unwell, and when I went to the loo I discovered I was bleeding. The floor manager followed me into the toilets. 'Are you OK, Bernie?' she asked kindly.

'No, I don't think I am. I'm bleeding.'

'OK, we'll get you to the hospital straight away.'

Neil insisted on driving me there himself and the floor manager came too, as someone from the crew had to be there for insurance purposes. We were all sitting in a row in the waiting-room at the hospital and people kept coming over to Neil and me, and saying, 'Oh, you two really are married!'

'Um, no we're not,' we kept mumbling, trying our best to smile politely.

Finally, I was taken into a cubicle for a scan and the sonographer said, 'Oh yeah, this isn't a viable pregnancy.'

What a terrible thing to say to someone! It seemed so cold.

'What do you mean, it's not viable?' I asked.

'You're having a miscarriage and you'll probably lose the pregnancy completely tomorrow.'

'Oh . . .' I went to the loo and had a cry, then I composed myself because I had to go back to the waiting-room and tell Neil. Poor Neil had found himself in the middle of my miscarriage, but he couldn't have been more supportive. He drove me home to Blackpool and he and his wife Deborah brought my car back from the studio the next day.

That morning I went to the loo and there it was in the toilet bowl – a tiny foetus. I told Steve I didn't want to flush it away for a few minutes and then I collapsed on to my knees and Steve caught me. Just then, Erin came into our dressingroom, which was next to the bathroom, and put her little arms around me.

'Don't worry, Mummy, she'll be with Kate now,' she said. 'She'll be OK.'

Erin was only a toddler at the time and we hadn't even told her I was having a baby – she must have overheard us talking. Her words literally took my breath away. 'If she can be that strong at her age, then I can, too,' I thought, getting up off the floor and wiping the tears from my eyes. My mum always said Erin was something special and that morning she proved it.

We were supposed to be moving into our new house that day – talk about bad timing – so Anne and Auntie Theresa came over and took Erin out for the day so Steve and I could finish packing.

I felt very low after the miscarriage, but I also appreciated how lucky I was to have Steve and Erin. The three of us were such a happy little team and I realised we didn't need another child to make our family complete. We decided not to try for more kids after that – Steve didn't want me to put myself through any more physical or emotional stress. And, to be honest, after going through what I did with Kate, neither did I.

On the positive side, I loved my job on *Brookside*. The cast – and the crew in particular – were amazing. They were like family, which helped when I had to film a miscarriage scene unnervingly similar to what had just happened to me for real. Everyone handled it really sensitively and the producer Paul was keen to make sure I was comfortable with it.

'Well, I've been through the real thing, so this will be nothing. It's just pretending,' I told him. But they were actually quite hard scenes to film, and I think Neil found them difficult, too. But we got through it.

After I'd been working on *Brookie* for a couple of years, my agent Tony got a call from Paul Marquess, who'd recently left the show to join ITV police drama *The Bill*. Apparently, he wanted me to come to London and join the cast of *The Bill*.

I was hugely torn, to be honest. *The Bill* was a prime-time show on ITVl but, on the other hand, I absolutely loved *Brookie* and all the people who worked on it. There had been lots of rumours, though, that *Brookside* was going to fold so, after lots of discussions with Steve and Tony, I decided not to renew my contract with *Brookside* and join *The Bill* instead.

My last scene was heartbreaking. I was splitting up with my husband Marty and had to say goodbye to my son in the show, who was played by Ray Quinn, who went on to be a huge success in *X Factor*, *Dancing on Ice* and on stage in the West End.

Neil and Ray were crying genuine tears and I could barely get my lines out.

'Hang on, I can't do this,' I said, sobbing. 'Look at Ray, he's got a big lip and he's sobbing! It's too hard.'

'Of course you can do it, Bernie,' said Neil. 'You're an actress. Just keep talking. It's real emotion, but it's good. Just get the words out.'

When we finished the scene everyone clapped and came over to give me a hug. God, it was so upsetting! I'd been very happy there. On the drive home to Blackpool that night I cried for the entire journey and all I kept thinking was: 'I really hope I'm doing the right thing.'

I was excited about joining *The Bill* though, and looking forward to getting stuck into my new role playing Sgt Sheelagh Murphy. I suggested to Steve that I could stay in London a couple of nights a week and commute back and forward to Blackpool the rest of the time, so that he and Erin wouldn't have to relocate, but he was dead against it. 'That's how marriages get into trouble,' he said. 'If you go, we all go.'

House-hunting in London was so depressing though! We loved our beautiful big Edwardian house, which we'd paid about £90,000 for, but we quickly discovered that kind of money wouldn't buy us a garden shed down South. Luckily, Linda stepped in and suggested we rented her friend's house in Hersham, Surrey, until we found something we could afford. It was a modern townhouse and, although it was lovely, it was absolutely tiny and felt really cramped compared to what we'd been used to.

Things were pretty challenging at first. Steve and I didn't know anyone in Hersham and had no friends or family living nearby – and we had a toddler. I was working all the hours that God sent – I'd leave the house at 5 a.m. and I'd get home at 9 p.m., and then I had to learn my scripts for the next day. It was knackering. Steve would make me some dinner while I memorised my lines, then I'd fall into bed exhausted. We weren't spending any proper time together.

Steve was doing everything at home – cooking, cleaning and looking after Erin. He went to mother and toddler groups with her, even though he was the only man. So, while I was out every day enjoying my new job and meeting lots of interesting people, Steve was stuck at home most of the day caring for Erin and he had no adult company until I came home at night. My mum couldn't come down to help out because she'd just been diagnosed with Alzheimer's and she wasn't up to it.

I started to dread coming home in the evenings because Steve was so moody. Sometimes I'd go for a drink with the cast rather than going straight home because I couldn't face arguing with him.

'What's the matter with you?' I snapped one night.

'Look, I haven't talked to an adult all day and now you're going on about your job, which is great, but I haven't got a job.'

It was obvious he was missing working and missing our life in Blackpool and, looking back, I can totally see why, but at the time we just rowed about it constantly.

'Why don't you just go home then?' I screamed at him one day. 'Why don't you go back to Blackpool?'

I knew then we needed to find our own place fast, somewhere with more space where Steve could have his drum kit and his keyboards and where we weren't living on top of each other.

We looked at sixty-two houses all over Surrey. Surrey was handy for *The Bill*, which was filmed in Merton at the time. Eventually, we found a house that we both fell in love with. It was in Weybridge, but it was on the market for a lot more money than we wanted to spend. Even though we'd sold our house up North and scraped together our savings, we were still £19,000 short for the deposit, so

Maureen's partner Ritchie lent us the rest of the money. I knew I'd be able to pay him back a few days later, which I did, when I received a cheque from a job I'd done. I was incredibly grateful to Ritchie because we would have missed out on the house if it hadn't been for his generosity. We still live in that house to this day.

Once we moved in, things started to get a lot better between Steve and me. We felt more relaxed in our own home and there was space for Erin to run around and for Steve to bring his equipment down from Blackpool.

Thank God, because I was genuinely worried we might split up when we were living in that little house in Hersham. We'd both admitted at different times that things weren't working and that we weren't happy, but we soldiered on because neither of us wanted to give up on the relationship. And I'm so glad we did. I think people give up on marriage too easily these days. It's hard being married sometimes and it's bloody hard being a new parent, so you have to work at it. We'd been through a lot in recent years – Kate's death, my dad dying and the miscarriage – but the move down South really tested us.

It worried me that I was so far away from Mum, too. When I phoned her for a chat, she'd always ask, 'What are you doing in London, Bernie?'

'I'm in *The Bill* Mum,' I'd say gently, over and over again.

'Oh, that's right,' she'd say. 'But what are you doing in London?'

Maureen used to say I was so patient with Mum, but of course I wasn't living in Blackpool like my brothers and sisters, who had to deal with the effects of the

Alzheimer's all the time, which must have been very upsetting and difficult. They all took turns having her to stay and I felt guilty that I wasn't able to help out more. But they all told me I'd be stupid to give up my job and not to worry, and I was grateful for their reassurance.

I did love *The Bill* and I was there for three years. The cast were great – brilliant folk like Kim Tiddy, John Bowler, Todd Carty and Trudie Goodwin. I also had an on-screen affair with Paul Usher, who'd previously played Barry Grant in *Brookside*. He was a mad Liverpool fan, so if there was a game on I'd sometimes find myself playing the scene to the floor manager while the camera focused in on me for a close-up. One time when a match was on, Paul ran out of the studio so quickly he smashed the glass in the doors!

My character also had an affair with Todd Carty's character PC Gabriel Kent, but when Todd decided he wanted to leave the show, it spelled the end for Sgt Sheelagh Murphy too. I don't think the show's execs could think of anywhere to go with my character, so I was called into a meeting one day and told they wouldn't be renewing my contract. I was upset about it, but instead of trying to save face by saying, 'I've told them I'm leaving,' I went into the canteen and announced to everyone that I'd been given the boot!

'OK, listen up everyone! I've been sacked! So it's goodbye from me and it's goodbye from her!'

Everyone just burst out laughing. Why lie about it? It was the truth and I didn't hold any grudges. I was determined to leave gracefully, and with my sense of humour intact. Yes, I was sad, but it's just the way things go – it's showbiz after all.

I wasn't sure what I was going to do work-wise – I just decided to see what came up. I figured that everything that had happened to me since I'd left the group had all been by chance. None of it had been planned, so I just hoped things would turn up.

Leaving *The Bill* enabled me to fulfil one of my long-held dreams – to make a solo album. I called it *All By Myself* and it's something I'm incredibly proud of to this day. Before, I'd never been happy with how I sounded on record because when the group was signed to CBS they always altered the speed of our tracks, which made me sound like a little girl. I chose all the tracks and arranged them all, too. I included a beautiful song called 'Better Place', which Steve wrote in memory of our daughter Kate.

Paul Muggleton produced the album and a guy called Matt Tate, who went on to work with Michael Jackson, mixed and mastered it, and I loved the way it sounded. David P Goods played guitar and also did a lot of the arrangements. One day I happened to tell Paul I'd love to do a duet with Peter Cox from Go West and he said, 'Oh, he's a friend of mine. I'll ask him.' I nearly dropped dead on the spot! So we did duet on a track called 'You Are Everything'. I was utterly gobsmacked by how good his voice was.

I'm so grateful to Paul for what he did on my album. I don't think he'll ever realise how important it was to me, to finally have something I could be proud of on record. It was released on a small independent label and there was no promotion so it didn't sell as well as it could have done, but I was just so glad I had the chance to do it. We had a lot of fun making that album, too. Paul is married to Judi Tzuke, a wonderful singer who had a massive hit called 'Stay With Me Till Dawn' in 1979, and Steve and I were huge fans. It was so lovely that we ended up spending some great times with Paul and Judi while I was making the record, sitting in their garden in the sunshine, drinking wine, laughing and chatting, and eating Judi's curry. It was wonderful.

In 2006 I was offered the chance to take part in a reality show called *The Games*. It involved competing against other celebrities in nine Olympic events, and we had to live together for ten days, so it was a bit like being in the *Big Brother* house. It required three or four months of training beforehand, but the money was really good – in fact, I would be earning the same weekly wage as I had been on *The Bill*. As the main breadwinner, I didn't feel I could turn it down. Plus, I was actually in really good shape because I'd made an exercise DVD called *40 and Fit for Life* while I was still in *The Bill*. I'd trained really hard and lost three stone, and I was super-fit and toned. How hard could it be? I hadn't quite taken into consideration the fact that I was forty-five at this point and most of the other people on the show were still in their twenties!

I hated it right from the word go, and when a car turned up at 4 a.m. to drive me to Nottingham in the snow so I could canoe on a frozen lake, I actually cried!

Steve told me to sod the money and pull out, but I hate letting people down, so I just told myself to stop being such a girl and get on with it. We had to learn how to roll ourselves under the water in a canoe in case we capsized when we were white-water rafting so, after breaking the ice on the lake, I took a deep breath and managed to tip myself under the icy water and come up again on the other side. But from that day on I was paralysed with fear and refused to do it again. It was freezing and pitch black under the water, and I hated it!

In the end they swapped the canoes for rafts, so if we fell out we'd just fall into the water and wouldn't risk being trapped in a canoe.

I had great fun with the other people on the show, though, especially Amanda Lamb, Michelle Gayle and Lib Dem MP Julia Goldsworthy. And I actually ended up finishing second in the rafting because Amanda and Julia both fell off!

Sports stars Sally Gunnell and Colin Jackson taught us hurdling, which was another ordeal for me because they don't alter the hurdles according to your height. So while Amanda, who's very tall, could practically step over the hurdles, they came right up to my waist because I'm only 5ft 1. It was pretty scary actually and Colin Jackson even told the bosses he was worried I'd break my leg. But, in the end, I jumped over every single hurdle and didn't knock one of them down. I came last, but at least I did it! I was so thrilled you'd have thought I'd won gold at the Olympics!

Every night we'd go back to the house and get drunk, which was hilarious. I was allowed to speak to Erin on the phone every night – I wouldn't have agreed to take part otherwise – and one night Steve came on the phone, 'Bernie, we're watching you now on the telly and I'm just ringing you to say stop . . .' and then he was cut off. He was trying to tell me I was making a show of myself, but I love to party and I was just having a good time. I wasn't doing anything really awful like stripping or farting! I was just being myself. So I ignored Steve, egged on by Amanda and Michelle of course!

On the last night I must admit I went to bed with a bottle of beer and made the girls laugh so much that Michelle fell out of bed and Amanda banged her head on the wall!

When we came out we had a wrap party and all the crew said the show would have been boring without me. Because I was older, I wasn't competitive at all. I didn't have a hope of winning, so I just decided to have a laugh. But one of the trainers told me that if I'd been the same age as the others I would have won, because I was incredibly fit for my age, so I was happy with that. Although I hated the events, the ten days I spent in the house turned out to be brilliant fun, so I was glad I'd stuck it out in the end.

In 2007 I joined the cast of a play called *Mum's the Word*, which is a great comedy piece a bit like *The Vagina Monologues*, with six women talking about the ups and downs of being a mum. I loved being back on stage again, so my manager Tony Clayman had an idea for a show called *Soap Queens* that I could do for the summer season in Blackpool alongside Debra Stephenson, who'd been in *Coronation Street*.

So that summer we did the Opera House every Sunday and opened the show singing 'Sisters Are Doin' It For Themselves'. Then we had a comedian on and Deborah, who's a gifted impressionist, did some comedy and I closed the second half with songs. We finished the show together singing 'Celebration' by Kool & the Gang.

It was a really good little show and the people who came to see it seemed to love it. Steve and I, and our mate Rick Coates, also put a band together called Hoops McCann and played gigs at the West Coast Rock Cafe, which is across the road from the Opera House. None of it earned us any real money but, after being on TV for the previous few years, it was nice to be singing in front of an audience again.

7
LOSING MUM

....

When my mum died just before Christmas 2007, it was a really strange feeling. I felt like we'd already lost her three or four years before when the Alzheimer's really took hold. She'd been deteriorating for years and it was truly heartbreaking to watch her regress to a childlike state. She would cry for no reason and shrink away from you as if you were a stranger, which I guess most of the time you were, and she even had to wear a nappy. She would sing 'Madame Butterfly' (her best song) at the top of her voice at three in the morning or she'd wander out of the house in the middle of the night and get lost. It was incredibly distressing. Luckily, the Nolans are so well known in Blackpool that someone would always bring her home safe.

It was such a huge strain on my brothers and sisters, who also had jobs and families to juggle, as well as caring for Mum. They all did their very best and I'm so proud of them. Eventually, though, we had to make the decision to put Mum into a home because it wasn't safe to leave her alone for any period of time.

Towards the end, she weighed about four and a half stone and only drank protein drinks through a straw. It was awful to see her looking so fragile and vulnerable. In December, Mum finally let go and passed away. It was so sad, but we were all relieved for her too. It's unbearable to see someone you love suffering so much.

I have a lovely memory of Mum from the last time I saw her, which will stay with me forever. It was about a month before she died and Maureen, Linda, Coleen and I went to see her at the home. We stroked her hair, kissed her and, I don't know why we did this as we never had before, but we started to sing her favourite songs. We sang 'The Sound of Music', 'Danny Boy' and 'Ireland, Mother Ireland'. We all cried and she actually looked up at us as if she was listening, and then she smiled at me. I was so touched by this little sign of recognition. It was a truly magical moment. I kissed and hugged her, and then we left. It was the last time I saw her.

For a long time afterwards I felt a lot of guilt about the fact that I lived in London when she was ill and didn't help out as much as the others, but none of my brothers and sisters ever made me feel bad about it. Maureen in particular always told me how patient I was with Mum, which I took great comfort from. Maureen has a knack of making everyone feel better – she's beautiful inside and out.

Then in 2008, just as we were getting over Mum's death, Anne announced that she was writing an autobiography and in it she was going to reveal that my dad had sexually abused her when she was a child. She'd actually told us about what Dad did to her a few years previously and we'd all been incredibly shocked and upset. Although I'd seen my dad's violent temper, I'd never ever seen that side of him. It explained a lot, though. Anne and Dad had always had a particularly difficult relationship and he was especially strict with her.

But when Anne called to warn me about the book, I told her I thought she ought to wait and publish it after Dad's sisters had died. Once Anne makes her mind up about something, though, there's no persuading her otherwise.

'I'm not phoning to ask your permission,' she said. 'I'm phoning to tell you it's happening.'

Understandably, Anne didn't have any regard for my dad, so she wasn't bothered about protecting his reputation, but I was concerned about his sisters, who were in their eighties at the time.

It's a big deal to go public with information like that and I suppose I felt there was something unfair about it because she wouldn't be hurting Dad – he was dead after all. That kind of thing affects so many other lives and her truth would hurt other people. So while I understood that writing the book might have been cathartic and have helped Anne to get closure, I also believed she should have waited.

It's not that I wasn't disgusted by what my dad did to Anne – I was. And I understood that people who have been victims of abuse often stay silent for years, as Anne had done, because they're too afraid to speak out. I was deeply, deeply shocked by the sexual aspects of my dad's behaviour, but it did seem to fit with his pattern of violence and need to exert authority. As a child, it had just felt like strict parenting, but with the benefit of hindsight, and looking at it through adult eyes, I can see how he fitted a certain profile, one that shocks and saddens me.

I believe my dad was sick to do what he did to Anne – the only way I can describe it is as a sickness – and yet I still love him. I'll never know or understand why he did what he did. Perhaps something happened in his own childhood, but whatever the case, there are no excuses. The only way I can look at it is to accept that some people's lives are screwed up and complicated, and you have to try to be forgiving.

It was very hard to reconcile the dad that I knew with the person who abused Anne. I remember watching Billy Connolly on TV, admitting that he still loved his late father, despite being sexually abused by him when he was a child, and it struck a chord with me. Although I accepted that what my dad did to Anne was very wrong and that he was an incredibly flawed character, I still loved him. It's a very hard thing to explain, but he was still my dad and had been a major figure in my life. We'd shared a passion for music and books, and I'd inherited his sense of humour, determination and love of performing. He was part of me and, whatever he'd done, that would never change.

I've always been very close to my sisters but I'd be lying if I said there wasn't rivalry between us girls – we're all in the same business and go for the same parts, but mostly we've been very supportive of each other. When

Denise didn't have any work, I gave her Bill Kenwright's number and told her to call him about the part of Mrs Johnstone and she ended up doing it for years. And it was Maureen who led me to my next part in the musical *Flashdance*.

We were doing *Mum's the Word* together when she mentioned she was going up for an audition for *Flashdance*.

'Damn, I should have gone up for that too,' I said.

'Oh, why don't you? I'll give you the producer's number,' she said, scrolling through the contacts list on her phone. 'Call him.'

So I did and I auditioned for the part of the mum – Hannah Owens – the day before Maureen.

'There's no point in me going now, is there?' laughed Maureen.

I did get the part and Maureen and I never rowed about it because it was all out in the open.

I ended up having a great time on *Flashdance*, which was adapted from the 1983 film of the same name. The tour kicked off in July 2008 at the Theatre Royal in Plymouth and it had a really successful run. There were some lovely people in the cast – Noel Sullivan, who'd started his career in the band Hear'Say after taking part in talent show *Popstars*, Bruno Langley, who'd played Todd Grimshaw in *Coronation Street*, and a wonderful singer and actress called Victoria Hamilton-Barritt, who played the lead, Alex Owens.

The travelling was pretty gruelling, though. We toured all over the UK for the next year and I did miss Steve and Erin a lot. I always tried to get home at the weekends and we'd spend every Sunday together and most of Monday, then I'd have to get in the car and drive to the next venue. It was very tiring but I loved my job.

8
FROM POP STAR TO OPERA STAR

....

At the start of 2009 I got a phone call from Maureen with some very big news.

'Bernie, we've been asked to do a Nolans reunion tour!' she squealed.

'Oh, my God, what's the story?' I blurted out, almost before she'd finished the sentence!

'Well, it would be with Live Nation and Universal, and they think it's perfect timing because this year is the thirtieth anniversary of "I'm in the Mood for Dancing". What do you think?'

'I think it sounds like a big deal!' I replied, already feeling excited.

Of course, we'd been asked to reunite for tours many times in the past, but it had never felt like the right time and we'd all been busy with other projects, plus we'd never been approached by companies as big as Live Nation and Universal before – they're huge in the entertainment business. So as soon as I heard they were involved, I knew it was an offer we had to take seriously.

Then when Coleen's manager Neil told me it was going

to be a nationwide theatre tour, taking in amazing venues such as the Hammersmith Apollo and the Liverpool Echo Arena, I immediately said, 'I'm in. Let's do it!'

The plan was for the tour to kick off in October, which was perfect timing for me. *Flashdance* was due to wrap up in the spring, which meant we could start rehearsals for the tour in the summer. I was absolutely thrilled that I had another great show to look forward to – with my sisters! I was on a real high.

But it wasn't long before I was brought crashing back to earth. I got a call from Neil to tell me it had been decided that Anne wasn't going to be involved in the tour. He explained that the bosses at Universal had decided they only wanted the four girls who were in the group when it was most successful, and that was Maureen, Linda, Coleen and me. Anne had left the group in 1980 and hadn't been around when we were at the height of our success. She'd sung on 'I'm in the Mood for Dancing', but she hadn't toured with us in Japan and Australia, and wasn't on our other big hits such as 'Gotta Pull Myself Together' and 'Who's Gonna Rock You?' But she had still been a big part of the group and I felt very upset that she was being left out. In fact, I was devastated for her and couldn't imagine how she must be feeling.

I talked to Maureen about it and we both agreed that Anne should be involved, so I called one of the bosses at Universal to try to convince her to rethink the line-up, but she wouldn't budge.

I consoled myself with the fact that Anne hadn't been in the business for a while. She'd been working for the tax office and seemed to love it, and I hadn't noticed any desire by her to go back to performing. 'Maybe she'll be OK with it,' I thought, optimistically.

But when I spoke to Anne on the phone, it was clear she was devastated. We had a lovely conversation, though, and before hanging up she said, 'Look, Bernie, give me a couple of weeks to get used to the idea and I'll be fine.'

I hoped things would be OK and that we could move on from it, but then Denise got involved maybe because she felt sorry for Anne. In the end, Anne started to feel that we ought to fight the decision instead of just accepting it. Sadly, after that things became more and more difficult.

The four of us who'd been asked to do the tour began getting texts from Denise, having a go at us for agreeing to perform without Anne, and all of sudden Anne was really upset. This all kicked off during the last couple of weeks of *Flashdance*, which was a real shame because I'd had a blast doing the show and it ruined the end of the tour for me. I was on my own in digs feeling really stressed and upset. I hated arguing with my sisters.

At first I tried to respond in a sensible way and explain that while I understood why they were upset, I'd already tried to talk to Universal about it, and now it looked like there was nothing more I could do. Denise and Anne thought that Maureen and I should pull out of the tour and force Universal to reconsider their decision. Universal wouldn't have any of that, though – in fact, they told us they would go ahead with the tour anyway with the majority of the lineup. Hearing that was a really horrible feeling.

If I'd been a millionaire, I might have turned it down but, to be brutally honest, I needed the cash. We were being offered an awful lot of money and I had to think about Erin and Steve – they were my priority now. I've always been very loyal to the group and to my family, but performing was my job, and there was no way I could justify saying no to the tour. Plus, I really wanted to do it. When Universal said they'd go ahead without Maureen and me, my heart sunk. I knew being on stage again with the other girls would be fantastic. It was an awesome opportunity.

I then got a text from Denise saying how disloyal I was, and that it seemed like the money was the only thing that was important to me, which was upsetting and very unfair. I realised Denise was sticking up for Anne, but in my opinion she went too far and made things worse. I hope that if she looked back now she'd agree.

All four of us felt ostracised – 'I've got no sisters now', Anne texted. I was distraught and kept texting back to ask what she meant. Of course I understood why she was upset, but the way she reacted really hurt me. Anne has had a lot to cope with over the years – the breakdown of her marriage, breast cancer and, of course, the abuse – and she'd dealt with everything with dignity.

But things just went from bad to worse when Anne, along with Denise and her partner Tom, threatened to sue us for the Nolan name. That actually made me laugh out loud. And it was such a shame because we'd come up with the idea of Anne guest appearing on a few of the tour dates – in our home town of Blackpool, for example. We could have been billed as 'The Nolans, featuring Anne Nolan'. But Universal got so fed up and wanted to avoid any controversy, and so as far as they were concerned it wasn't an option.

By this point I'd started to feel really angry. I felt I'd tried to get Denise to see my point of view, but eventually I said, 'This is ridiculous. I'm not going to text you any more. You've disowned us anyway, so that's the end of it'. I just stopped replying to her texts and Anne changed her number, so we couldn't communicate with her anyway.

I think Denise's view is that if you're family, you stick together no matter what, but I don't agree with that. Family aren't always right just because they're family and if I believe someone is wrong, I'll say so.

It was an awful time and it's still awful because Coleen doesn't talk to Anne and Denise now. It was terrible for Maureen in particular, as she lives just around the corner from Anne and Denise in Blackpool. The three of them had always been so close – they were inseparable. I was sad about what happened, mostly because of how it affected Maureen. If I'd been left out of the tour, I would have been upset too, but I like to think I would have dealt with it differently. However bad I'd felt, I would have wished the other girls good luck and I'd have been in the front row cheering them on – my pride wouldn't have allowed me to do anything else.

Although it was upsetting that we were at loggerheads with Anne and Denise, we had to push it to the backs of our minds because we were about to start rehearsals for the show.

Maureen and I had been working away at our solo

careers, but Coleen hadn't sung live for about seventeen years and the four of us hadn't performed on stage together for a quarter of a century!

To be honest, there were a few tensions to begin with because we were all vying for our place in the band. The only thing we'd ever rowed about was our act – what we were going to sing and what we were going to wear. We may share family traits, but we all have very different personalities. And having been a solo artist for a long time it was difficult for me to slip back into that group mentality. In the past, I'd hated not being able to say what I thought – it always had to be The Nolans' opinion and I was always getting into trouble with the rest of them for speaking out of turn! It was hard to be individual.

Musically, we never agreed on anything and I was always outvoted. When we took a vote on something and it ended up two against two, it was like a fight to the death! Coleen is very laidback so she'd often say, 'I don't mind . . . whatever,' which is lovely in one way, but in another way it's a nightmare because I'd be thinking, 'Make a decision!' And when Anne was in the group we used to row a lot because we're both such strong characters with completely different views on life and music.

The four of us decided to go to Coleen's house in Cheshire to start working on the music for the tour. I realise I'm quite exacting when it comes to music, which can probably be annoying. Of course I like to have a laugh, but I like to get the work done as well and I enjoy the rehearsal process. I began to think the others weren't taking it quite as seriously as I was. There was a lot of messing about, a lot of talking and a lot of cups of tea!

I remember one weekend we rehearsed all day, then went out for a meal and a few drinks in the evening, and ended up having an almighty row. I was explaining to Coleen that we needed to take things more seriously and stop wasting time, but I felt like the three of them then ganged up on me. 'You're so pedantic,' 'You think you know it all,' 'We need to have fun, too!' they were all saying.

I don't know who was right or wrong, but what hurt me was that it got personal. It started off as a minor disagreement over messing about in rehearsals, but then it snowballed and things were said between us that had been simmering for years. It eventually got very hurtful for all concerned and I ended up in tears.

I felt that there had always been a little bit of underlying tension and animosity in the group because I'd sung lead vocals on all our hits, but that hadn't been my choice. The way it worked was that we all had to sing the track, almost like an audition, and then the producer had usually ended up picking me. But the girls hadn't complained at the time. We'd all wanted to have hits and the producers felt I had the most commercial pop voice.

But later that night after the bust up, I just couldn't sleep, so I called Steve and asked him what I should do. He advised me to stick it out and said things would be fine, but I just wanted to go home, so I booked a taxi and train for the next day.

When I came downstairs with my suitcase in the morning, the girls were all really shocked.

'Where are you going?' asked Maureen, looking worried.

'I'm going home where I'm loved and respected, because I don't feel that here,' I shot back.

'But you can't go home, Bernie. We're meant to be rehearsing today,' she pleaded.

But this time I wasn't having any of it.

'You might be rehearsing, but I'm not. I'm an adult and I can do what I like! I know my parts anyway,' I replied, which I'm sure didn't go down well because it sounded bigheaded!

As I was getting my things together to leave, Maureen said, 'Come here,' and gave me a big hug. She's so soft! She was trying to be strong and be the big sis, but ended up sobbing on my shoulder.

I went home and had a lovely weekend with Steve and Erin, then went back to Coleen's on Monday to rehearse. I just had to get out, get over it and regroup and things were fine from then on. We carried on as if nothing had happened, and although things got off to a rocky start, we ended up having a great laugh that summer.

But when it comes down to it, I know my sisters are my biggest fans. In fact, Maureen is like a window licker! She comes to see me wherever I'm performing and they're all really proud of me. In the group, though, I did feel a bit of pressure because I was singing everything and I think it was a case of old tensions resurfacing.

As the tour drew closer, our excitement began to mount. There was about £2 million behind the production, so we had fabulous sets and eight dancers. In the old days things were much more basic – we had our own band and a lighting rig, but that was pretty much it. We even organised our stage outfits and did our own make-up, so this tour was in another league entirely.

For me, the best thing was having the luxury of professional stylists and hair and make-up artists. All we had to think about was getting to the gig, where our costumes were hanging neatly on rails and baskets of freshly laundered underwear were waiting for us in our dressingrooms, then we'd be pampered for three hours before the show – pure bliss!

Each of our songs had a dance routine, choreographed by Kim Gavin, who was my producer on *Flashdance*. Kim had choreographed tours for Take That and went on to be the creative director for the 2012 Summer Olympics Closing Ceremony, so we were thrilled to get the opportunity to work with him for the tour.

Before we went on the road, our entire set was put up at a studio in Elstree for a dress rehearsal in front of an invited audience, mostly made up of family and friends. It was so exciting! We'd rehearsed for four days solidly prior to the performance and it paid off because we did the whole show without stopping and got an amazing reaction from the crowd. We were ready!

Straight after the Elstree run-through, we all piled on to a coach to travel to Nottingham for our opening night on 11 October 2009. I remember noticing how fit and healthy I felt – perhaps it was down to all the dancing I'd been doing in rehearsals – and I was looking forward to throwing myself into the tour.

The first night at the Royal Concert Hall in Nottingham was nerve-wracking, though, because I desperately wanted it to be good. Coleen's sons, Shane Junior and Jake, were our support act and, to be honest, I was a little worried about that because they'd never performed live together and I hadn't even heard them sing before. But they were absolutely fantastic and perfect for our crowd because the women loved them!

I was in the dressingroom getting ready when I heard the music for their first song come on – Take That's 'Greatest Day' – and then a huge roar from the crowd. Coleen and I had a little peek from behind the scenes and saw the theatre was already packed. With each song, the cheers got louder and there were even people up dancing. Usually there isn't a full house for the support act, but because Coleen's kids were opening the show, the place was rammed. We were all so proud of the boys and they loved it too.

Then it was time for us to go on! I had butterflies, but I also felt well prepared – I knew my harmonies, I knew my choreography and the beautiful make-up and glamorous outfits definitely gave me an extra confidence boost. For our opening number we wore black high-waisted trousers with a sequinned unitard underneath and a white tux jacket over the top.

We started the show at the top of a staircase behind a big screen, which pulled back when the music started to reveal the four of us, standing with our backs to the audience. An almighty cheer went up from the crowd when they saw us and I was desperate to turn round to the other girls and mouth, 'Oh my God!' but we had to stay in position. I wanted to scream and cry all at the same time – it was one of the best feelings ever and something I'll never forget. When we turned round to break into our version of Bonnie Tyler's 'Hero', the entire place was on its feet. Women were waving feather boas and singing along.

Although we knew the tickets had sold well, I suppose at the back of my mind I was worried that people wouldn't turn up because the group had been out of the limelight for so long. So to see the crowd enjoying themselves so much was amazing.

We all performed solo numbers during the show – Coleen sang Alesha Dixon's 'The Boy Does Nothing', Linda sang Duffy's 'Mercy', Maureen did 'Valerie' by The Zutons and I sang 'So What' by Pink.

All the dates on the tour were brilliant, but the opening night was really special – it couldn't have been better. There was a real party atmosphere, which is exactly what we'd hoped for. When we were doing our promotion for the show, the message we wanted to get across to women was, OK, life can be dull sometimes and when you've had kids you often wonder if you'll do anything for yourself ever again, so get your glad rags on, have a glass of wine and come along to our show to party with us. And boy, did they come in their droves!

There was a lot of drunkenness going on in some of the venues, too. One night a massive fight broke out at the back of the crowd. We'd actually cut back on security because we didn't think we'd need it at a Nolans gig. And I always hated it when the security guys stopped fans from shaking our hands. We wanted to meet people and we wanted everyone up dancing, but the other venues heard about this fight and some of them got really strict, and wouldn't allow dancing. Of course, we'd tell the audience, 'Ignore these guys. Stand up and dance!'

At one venue, a woman jumped up on stage and headed

straight for me, which was kind of scary, but she just wanted to hug me really.

The whole experience was amazing – every night when that screen went back the roar from the crowd was deafening. In some ways I felt we'd never got the credit we deserved all those years ago, so this tour was saying 'Fuck you!' to all those people who'd taken the mickey out of us! I'm sure some people did come along to laugh at us, but when they saw us perform they thought, 'Hmm, they're actually really good and they can sing live.'

The other lovely thing about the tour was that it was a real family affair. Steve was playing drums in our band, Coleen's husband Ray was on guitar, Ciara was on the road with us and, of course, Shane and Jake were supporting us.

I hate taking Erin out of school – I'm a very strict mum when it comes to that – but she joined us on the tour during her half-term holiday in October, which we extended by another week with permission from her school. It broke my heart when we had to leave her behind at Elstree after the warm-up show and she was crying as we pulled away in the coach, which of course meant I was in floods of tears too. But I knew she'd be taken care of wonderfully by our friends Sue and Duncan, who she stayed with for most of the time Steve and I were away.

The following night, though, we got a call to say Erin was really ill with a sore throat and a temperature. I was so worried about her, but she asked to speak to me and said, 'I'm not very well, Mum, but don't worry, I'll be OK. I'm sitting here watching DVDs. Just enjoy yourself and I hope it goes great.' She was amazing – and only ten years old at the time. I have to say at this point that I really lucked out having Erin as a daughter because she's always been such a mature and sensible girl, and I'm incredibly proud of her.

And when she did get to come on tour with us, she had a ball. She's crazy about dancing, so she'd sit at the back of the coach with all the dancers and I hardly saw her. I was at the front with Steve and the other boys from the band, and my sisters sat in the middle part of the coach. We did lots of quizzes on the tour bus to stop boredom setting in and Erin read out the questions over the mic. Then at Halloween we were in Sheffield and she dressed up with the dancers and we had a big party in our hotel bedroom. She had a lot of fun and she'll remember all of those good times, and will hopefully be able to look back on a wonderful childhood.

I'm so glad we did the tour, despite all the rows with Anne and Denise, because it was one of the best things I've ever done in my life. And I did think of Anne. On many occasions I thought, 'If Anne were here now she'd love this'. But sadly it had been out of my hands.

The tour wound up on 10 November at the Belfast Odyssey and although I really wanted to take some time off to be at home with Steve and Erin, I had to go into rehearsals for panto in Dunstable almost straight away. I had enough money that year not to have to do panto, but I'd signed up for it before we were offered the tour. So after being on the road for weeks I had to work all over the Christmas holidays too.

Now and Forever

I was playing the Fairy Godmother in *Cinderella* opposite Basil Brush, so in the blink of an eye I'd gone from singing to thousands of people to dancing around a puppet – that's how bizarre show business can be. It was a great panto though, and the kids loved Basil!

Christmas day in Weybridge was quiet but lovely – just Steve, Erin and me, and our two friends Drew and Grant. On reflection, it had been a great year, but incredibly busy, so although I missed seeing my relatives over the holidays it was nice to spend the little time off I had just chilling out at home.

At the start of January, while I was still in panto, I noticed my left breast looked a bit odd. I'd stripped off to get into the shower one morning and caught sight of myself in the bathroom mirror. My breast looked a little dimpled underneath and when I lifted up my arm I could see the dimpling more clearly.

When I got out of the shower, I showed Steve. 'Does that look weird to you?' I asked, pointing to the dimpled area.

'Umm, not really,' he replied.

To be brutal, when you get to my age, cellulite starts popping up in all sorts of unexpected places, so I didn't think that much of it at the time. I did have a feel to check for lumps, but I didn't find anything and I certainly didn't immediately think I might have cancer. Physically, I felt fine and assumed the dimpling was probably just down to getting older, so I put it to the back of my mind and made a mental note to see the doctor as soon as I got the chance.

When panto finished, there was another big project just around the corner. In December Coleen's agent Neil Howarth had called me to ask if I was interested in taking part in a new show that was coming on in the New Year. It was called *Popstar to Operastar* and would feature a group of pop and rock singers turning their hand to more traditional music. 'So, would you like to be considered for it?' Neil asked. 'I'd love to,' I replied. I'm so passionate about singing and this was a chance to learn a whole new vocal skill that was out of my comfort zone. So when he rang at the start of the year to tell me I'd got the gig, I was thrilled. The only problem for me was that the job had come through Coleen's agent, who had organized the tour. It meant I was going to have to leave my old agent, Tony, whom I'd worked with since I was in The Nolans. He was a great guy, and I adored him and his family, but I felt I had to move on.

The show kicked off in mid January and I loved it from day one. I never realised I had that sort of voice. My mum always said, 'You could be a soprano, Bernie,' when I was just messing about, singing around the house. But when I started rehearsing for the show, the singing coaches all told me I was a natural soprano. Mum was right after all! I thought I knew a lot about singing, but the show taught me so much about breathing and technique. It was wonderful.

Classical stars Katherine Jenkins and Orlando Villazón were our mentors, but we also had fantastic singing teachers called Claire Moore and Mary King. And my fellow contestants were lovely, too – Danny Jones from McFly, Vanessa White from The Saturdays, Jimmy Osmond,

Kym Marsh, Marcella Detroit from Shakespears Sister, Alex James from Blur and Darius Campbell, who'd found fame on *Pop Idol*.

Everyone was incredibly nervous – it was terrifying having to sing opera live in a foreign language – so the first week I suggested we all went to the pub across the road for dinner to take our minds off the performance. So we did, and every week after that a few of us went to the pub and had a laugh, which really helped to combat the nerves.

The show was recorded on a Friday, so we'd spend all day at the studio for rehearsals, then we'd get our hair and make-up done and flowers would arrive in our dressing-rooms with good luck messages. And I got to wear the most fabulous costumes – long flowing evening dresses and beautiful ball gowns. One week they gave me a man's song so I wore a tux, which was fun.

Steve and Erin always came to see me. I'd promised Erin she could have a new dress for every week I managed to stay in the show, which ended up costing me a fortune because I was there till the end!

After the show we'd all go for drinks in the bar, so it was lots of fun. I remember saying to Steve, 'What the hell are we going to do on Fridays when this is all over?'

On the last night it was down to Darius, Marcella and me, and we got to choose what to sing. I chose 'Les Filles de Cadix', which is a pretty challenging song, but Darius beat me by half a point and I had to make do with runner-up.

Everyone in the studio that night was convinced I was going to win the competition, so it was a bit of a shock all round when Darius's name was read out. The green room was buzzing with my friends and family who all thought I was going to win it. And I was close! I found out later I'd won the public vote every week apart from the first one.

Everyone said I should have performed 'Parla Più Piano' – the theme from *The Godfather* – which the crowd went crazy about when I'd sung it on week two, but I wanted to do something more difficult to demonstrate how much I'd progressed on the show. Typical me to go for the harder option!

But you can't look back with regret. I do think that my improvement from beginning to end was a much bigger leap than Darius's, but that's showbiz! It's mostly women who vote on these shows, and Darius is a good looking guy as well as being a great singer. Still, I'm not bitter. I'd had an absolutely brilliant time and I wouldn't have missed it for the world.

In February, towards the end of *Popstar to Operastar*, the dimpling on my breast started to play on my mind. I still couldn't find a lump, but I noticed the area around my nipple felt different. It felt hard. I'd signed up to do a tour of *Mum's the Word*, which kicked off in Bradford at the beginning of April, so I decided to see my GP before things got too crazy again with work. My back had been bothering me, so I needed to get that seen to anyway, and I thought I'd ask about my breast at the same time.

I was actually standing up to leave the surgery when I said: 'Look, I know you're supposed to come here with one complaint at a time, but while I'm here I'd like you to have a look at my left breast because it looks as if it's changed – it's a bit dimply.'

'OK, I'll check it out,' he said, gesturing for me to sit back down.

'I can't feel a lump though, so it's probably just me being silly,' I added apologetically, as he began to examine me.

'Oh, I can feel a lump,' he said.

But even when he guided my hand to where the lump was, I still couldn't feel it. I was shocked and my first thought was, 'Oh, shit, here we go.' Naturally, I was concerned because there's a history of breast cancer in our family – Anne and Linda had both battled it in recent years and, thankfully, had beaten it. But I told myself there was no point in worrying until I knew for sure that there was something to worry about.

My doctor made an appointment for me to have a mammogram on 12 April at a breast-screening clinic in Guildford called the Jarvis Centre, which meant I had a week to wait before there was any more information.

I went home and told Steve, who was as shocked as I was, but we're quite pragmatic as a couple and decided the only thing to do was to carry on as normal until I'd been for the mammogram. I'm very positive by nature and I've never seen the point in wasting my life worrying about things that haven't happened yet. So I carried on with *Mum's the Word*, which was perfect because it meant I didn't have time to dwell on anything for too long. And Steve and I really didn't discuss it much over the next few days.

On the day of the mammogram I was a little apprehensive

but not worried. I'd had mammograms in the past and although they're uncomfortable, just as you're thinking, 'If they squeeze this breast any more it's going to pop!' it's all over.

Steve came to the appointment with me and sat in the waiting-room while I had the mammogram. Usually, once it's been done, you wait for a few minutes, then you're told it's OK for you to go home. After I'd been seen I was chatting to Steve in the waiting-room. I remember we were laughing about something silly when the nurse popped her head around the door. 'Bernie, can you hang around?' she asked.

As soon as I heard those words I knew something must be wrong. I started to get butterflies, but before I had a chance to say anything to Steve, I was called back into the screening room.

'Bernie, we can see a lump on the scan and we'd like to do a needle biopsy now,' said the nurse gently.

'We've also detected a lot of calcium in your breast and that's a sign of breast cancer to come,' she added.

I felt numb with shock. 'OK,' I nodded, slowly taking off my top and bra so they could perform the biopsy. I had an injection to freeze the area first, but the procedure was still incredibly painful and I cried.

As I was getting dressed, the nurse said, 'We have to send this sample of tissue away to be tested, but I do this every day and I believe you do have breast cancer. We don't make mistakes.'

I felt sick and overwhelmed, and that's when I said, 'I don't want to die,' and the tears started to fall. I'd been trying so hard not to cry, which is sad in itself.

'One step at a time, Bernie,' said the nurse reassuringly. 'Let's not run before we can walk.'

She was absolutely lovely. We take people like her for granted, but how do you tell someone that kind of news?

'Would you like me to tell your husband?' she asked.

'Yes, I'll go and get him,' I said.

Steve was reading a magazine in the waiting-room, completely unaware that I was about to shatter his world. I stood and looked at him for a few seconds, delaying that moment when I called him into the room because I knew when I did that our lives would never be the same.

'Steve, you'd better come in,' I said, beckoning him over.

The nurse was wonderful with him. 'You're probably wondering why we've been so long, Steve,' she said. 'When we did the mammogram we could see a lump, so we decided to do a biopsy, which we're sending off to be tested, but as I explained to Bernie, in my view it looks very much like breast cancer.'

I glanced up at Steve and saw he'd gone deathly pale. It was awful to see him like that.

'You'll get the results in a week but, as I've told Bernie, we don't make mistakes here,' she added.

I appreciated her honesty and that she didn't want to send us away with false hope.

'What would you like to do? You're welcome to sit here for a while,' she said, getting up to pour us some water.

'So what happens now?' I ventured.

'Once we get the results we'll decide on a plan. I know it's hard, but try not to think too far ahead.'

I just couldn't believe it. I'd always associated lumps with cancer, but this was just a bit of dimpling. I'd seen my doctor within eight weeks of realising my nipple felt different, but I would have gone sooner if I'd known about the other signs of breast cancer. I know now through Breakthrough Breast Cancer's TLC (Touch, Look, Check) campaign that there are several other signs besides lumps, including dimpling of the skin and changes to the nipple. But, of course, you never imagine it will happen to you. I felt healthy and had as much energy as ever, and it didn't enter my head that the orange-peel skin underneath my breast could mean I had cancer.

Steve and I walked out of the breast-screening clinic in silence, holding hands, but when I got into the car I absolutely broke down and cried my eyes out. Steve just held me tight and kept repeating, 'You'll be fine, Bernie. You'll be here forever. Nothing's going to happen to you.' I'm not sure if he was trying to convince me or himself. I think he was still in shock.

I really let off steam in the car. I felt shocked and devastated and angry. I was most upset when I started thinking about what this meant for Erin and the impact it could have on her life. She was so young and I instantly wanted to protect her from what was happening. My mind was racing. How could we tell her? How would she take it? I couldn't bear the thought of dropping this bombshell into her life. I remember shouting, 'Shit! I can't believe I've done this to Erin and that I'm bringing this into our house,' which made Steve angry because he didn't want me blaming myself.

'Don't say that! It's not your fault,' he said.

I must have cried solidly for five minutes and then I just stopped.

'Right, that's it!' I said, drying my eyes with a tissue and reaching for my seatbelt. We had to get going to be home in time for Erin.

'I've done my thing. Let's get on with it. We've just got to deal with it, Steve. We don't know the full story yet, so let's keep it to ourselves for now and just try to be normal if we can.'

I'm not sure where that steely attitude came from, but it set the tone for how I'd be over the next few months. And what was the alternative – to lock myself in a room and wait to die? I didn't know what the future held, but I did know I had a wonderful life and a husband and a daughter who loved me. I had it all to live for.

9
THE BATTLE BEGINS

....

It was the Easter holidays and Steve and Erin were due to come with me to Lincoln where *Mum's the Word* was opening. We decided to stick to our plans because we wanted to keep things as normal as possible for Erin. Plus, there was nothing we could do back in London until we had the diagnosis confirmed.

I tried my best not to dwell on what had happened at the breast-screening centre, but of course it was hard. Fortunately, work kept me busy and because Erin was with us, we had to think up ways of keeping her occupied. Lincoln is a lovely place and our digs were great so, despite the circumstances, we tried to make the best of it.

Then, towards the end of the week, I got a phone call from a breast care nurse at the Royal Surrey County Hospital.

'Mrs Doneathy, I'm sorry to tell you that the tests have confirmed what we thought. It is breast cancer,' she said.

'Right, thanks,' I replied, immediately thinking how funny it was that I'd just thanked her for telling me I had breast cancer.

'We'll let you know about your next appointment soon and what's going to happen next,' she continued.

Although I'm the sort of person who always tries to see the positive in every situation, I'm a realist too. Of course I'd been hoping that some terrible mistake had been made and that I just had a harmless cyst, but deep down I knew there wouldn't be any other outcome.

After that, things began to happen very quickly. Within a week of the phone call I was sent to the Royal Surrey for my first appointment with a lovely breast care nurse called Helen. What I liked about Helen was that she was very matter-of-fact – not in a horrible way, but she gauged my personality just right. I don't mind a hug, but I didn't want pity or sympathy and all that 'Oh, you're so brave!' rubbish, and she picked up on that straight away.

'Right, what's the next stage? What do we have to do?' I asked her.

'Well, you know the situation, you know it's breast cancer, so you'll have the lump removed, but because there's a lot of calcium in the breast, we'd definitely recommend a mastectomy,' she said, pointing to my scan.

'That will turn into breast cancer, so even if you had the lump removed, the cancer would come back.'

'Oh, OK.' I hadn't really thought about having my breast removed.

The next step, Helen told me, was to decide which surgeon I wanted to do the procedure. She gave me a booklet, which in hindsight I wish she hadn't given me. It had pictures of the surgery in brutal detail.

'A lot of women like to see this, so they're prepared for what's going to happen and how they'll look,' she said.

'Oh, really? I'm not sure,' I said, closing it quickly.

'Well, take it. You don't have to look if you don't want to. Your consultant will explain anyway.'

I actually didn't want to know what was going to happen to me in that much detail. I was happy to let the experts do their thing while I was asleep!

After that first appointment I had another cry in the car when Steve and I were on our way home from the hospital. I guess the reality of what I was about to face started to hit home.

'I'm not going to cry any more,' I said to Steve once I'd calmed down. And apart from one particularly low moment during my chemo, I didn't. I'm a very determined and optimistic person, and right from the word go I decided to deal with cancer head on and to try really hard not to let it beat me. Of course I accepted my life was going to change, but I didn't want to ruin what life I might have left by being constantly depressed. I didn't know I'd react like that – I could have fallen to pieces, but my attitude was always, 'I'm living with this, not dying from it.'

And I had Erin to think about. I still wanted her life to be great. I didn't want to ruin her life or Steve's. I felt my attitude was crucial to how they coped with my illness. If I'd started off being negative, everyone else would have reacted the same way. And what would be the point in making everyone's life miserable?

I decided on a surgeon called Mark Kissin. As surgeons go, he's like God at the Royal Surrey! 'He hasn't got a great bedside manner,' Helen warned me. 'But he has a wonderful reputation and he's a brilliant surgeon.'

He'd performed hundreds of these procedures and he would be able to do the reconstruction at the same time, which appealed to me. I didn't relish the idea of going back months later for more surgery. And I wanted to wake up and still have both breasts – mentally I thought that would be easier to deal with. Also, if there was no cancer in my nipple, I'd be able to keep it, which is quite rare.

When I met Mr Kissin I liked him right away – he's straight-talking like me, and has quite a serious manner like Steve. He tells it like it is, which is exactly what I was after.

'How are you doing today?' he asked, gesturing for Steve and me to sit down.

'I'm fine,' I chirped.

'You're fine? Good, that's all I need to know.'

Mr Kissin went on to explain that I had HER2 positive breast cancer, which is an aggressive form of the disease. He wanted me to have chemotherapy straight away to stop it spreading instead of waiting until after the mastectomy, which is usually the case. He said my oncologist would be Dr Stephen Houston – 'One of the best in the country,' he assured me.

On the plus side – if there is such a thing – the three tumours I had were very small. Mr Kissin told us what the surgery would involve and that he'd take muscle from my back for the reconstruction. I suggested that maybe he should take off both breasts just to be on the safe side.

'Hang on a second. One thing at a time,' he said calmly. 'We don't need to take the other breast – the scan doesn't show any calcium in it, but we'll do a biopsy while you're under, just to double-check.

'There's a chance it could have spread to your lymph nodes, but we'll take some out while you're on the operating table and test them there and then.'

It was a lot to take in, but I felt reassured that there was a plan of action and I was keen to start the treatment as soon as possible. But what was I going to do about work? I was still in *Mum's the Word*. I explained to Mark that I was touring and had to drive every Monday to different venues, stay in digs and lug my suitcase up and down stairs.

'Well, people do carry on working,' he said. 'You should just listen to your body.'

'But what would be better for her, Mark?' Steve chipped in. 'Would it be better for her to be at home with no stress and no driving?'

'In my opinion it would be better if she wasn't working because then all her energy would go into the fight.'

I didn't need any more convincing. I wanted to fight this disease with every fibre of my being. How could I do that if I was devoting so much energy to being on stage every night? I love performing live, but it can be a stressful thing and it's very demanding, both physically and mentally.

After the meeting with Mark I called Robert Kelly – the producer of *Mum's the Word* and also a friend – and explained I'd been diagnosed with breast cancer and wouldn't be able to finish the tour. I said I didn't know how the chemo would affect me and I didn't want to mess him around by being off work all the time.

When I'd finished my little speech, he said, 'Look Bernie, nothing is more important than your health. Go and get yourself better and this role will always be here for you.'

He was amazing. Show business can be cruel and cutthroat, and a lot of producers wouldn't have been like that. Some of them might have threatened to sue me! It happens. But Robert didn't put any pressure on me at all, which was just what I needed.

We still hadn't told Erin at this point. It was her birthday on 26 April – she was turning eleven – and I wanted to wait until after that. But Erin had other plans. We picked her up from school after our meeting with Mr Kissin. I told her I'd been attending a well woman clinic, but she wasn't buying it. We were sitting in the living-room, reading and watching telly before dinner, when Erin suddenly piped up, 'What's up with you two?' Kids are very intuitive, right?

'I know there's something wrong; I know there is,' she insisted.

'What do you mean, darling?' I asked.

'I know there's something wrong because Dad's being extra, extra nice to you. He's always kissing you and, I don't know, he just seems weird. You'd better tell me, Mum.'

So I looked at Steve and he looked at me, and I thought, 'Well, we're going to have to tell her.' She was aware that something was going on and I didn't want her imagining an even worse scenario. I got up and sat next to her and said, 'Look, Erin, I haven't been to a well woman clinic. I've been to see a doctor because I've got breast cancer.'

Before I had a chance to say anything else, she immediately came back with, 'Are you going to die?'

'No, I'm not going to die! Look at Auntie Anne and Auntie Linda – they're both fine now.'

Because cancer has been in our family, it's perhaps not such a scary word and it was great to be able to use my sisters as proof that you can beat it.

'I've got to have a mastectomy and they'll get it all out, then I'll be on chemotherapy for a while, so I might lose my hair,' I explained. 'I might be tired or feel ill sometimes, but we'll just deal with each thing as it comes along. But I'm not going to die, Erin.'

One little tear trickled down her cheek, just one, and she said, 'OK, I don't want to talk about it any more.'

'That's fine,' I said. 'You don't have to talk about it at all, but if you have any questions, you just have to ask. Shall we find a different name for it, though?'

Her eyes lit up. 'Yeah. I think because it begins with C it ought to be Celia,' she said.

'Oh my God, why? I have a friend called Celia and she's not going to be happy!' I said.

'That makes it even funnier,' she giggled. Erin has a great sense of humour, just like her dad, and it helped lighten the mood after a very tough day.

Of course my friend Celia wasn't too thrilled when I told her. 'No disrespect! It's nothing to do with you,' I assured her!

I was massively relieved that Erin took the news OK. When you're facing something as scary and life-changing as cancer, being a parent is the hardest thing. I felt so guilty because I'd brought cancer into her world. Illness, chemo, medication and hospital visits would inevitably become part of her life too, and become part of her childhood memories. I felt very angry about that.

On the positive side, kids give you the strength to keep

fighting and they provide a wonderful sense of normality. Life goes on for them because it has to. Just being a mum and doing all the usual stuff for Erin really helped me.

I realised long before I had cancer that I'd been given the most brilliant child, but it really hit home after my diagnosis. I'm not religious at all, but my mum was, and after I had Erin she said, 'She's an angel that child. She's been sent to you from God because you lost Kate.'

'What do you mean, Mum?' I asked.

'I don't know, there's just something special about her,' she said. And there is.

I know everyone thinks their child is special and everyone's child is special, but the way Erin has coped with things is extraordinary. In fact, she was coping so well after I told her about the breast cancer that I worried she was in denial, but I asked a few of her friends and their parents how she behaved when I wasn't around and they all told me she was handling things really well.

Erin's attitude helped me more than words can say and I thank God for her every day because it could have been so much worse. I still made sure I asked her every couple of weeks how she was feeling though. I've always tucked her into bed at night – I scratch her back and sing to her as she's drifting off to sleep, so I'd wait until bedtime, when it was just the two of us, and say softly, 'How are you doing with everything? Have you got any questions?'

She'd always reply, 'No, Mum! If I've got questions, I'll ask you.' She's very practical, which is a trait she inherited from me.

'OK, well that's great, but you can ask me or your dad anything.'

'Yeah, I know,' she'd say, before moving on to something else. I remember once she asked if the cancer meant we couldn't go to Maureen's wedding in Spain, which was planned for August. Steve thought it was selfish of Erin to be worried about missing out on a holiday, but I thought it was great! It meant she was acting like a normal kid and that's what I wanted.

Her eleventh birthday provided a little ray of sunshine in what had been one of the darkest months of our lives. She had some friends round for a sleepover the weekend before, then on the Monday, which was her birthday, we went to a restaurant with our friends Sue and Duncan, who live round the corner, and their two kids, James and Rachel. We had balloons and presents piled high on the table, and I'd hired a Harry Potter lookalike to do magic tricks. Erin absolutely loved it and, despite everything that was going on, it was a great birthday.

'I don't want to think about cancer on my birthday, Mum,' she said to me quietly.

'No, neither do we, Erin,' I reassured her. 'You don't need to think about it at all.'

There's no upside to cancer, but one thing it did give me was the opportunity to spend more time at home with Erin because I'd given up work. I could be there for her 24/7, which was wonderful. I loved just doing normal mum things at home – it was a revelation! And it was a relief not to have to pack my bags on a Sunday night and go on tour.

But while Erin was pretty stoic, Steve reacted differently. For a couple of weeks after my diagnosis, he struggled to cope. He just couldn't handle the thought of me not being there. He always thought I'd live forever. In fact, he often said, 'You'll live forever, you!' probably because I take after my Auntie Lily, who lived to be ninety-nine and still enjoyed a drop of whisky and loved a little dance right up until she passed away. She was amazing. 'That'll be you,' Steve would joke.

I'm sure a lot of people used to think of me in that way, maybe because I've always been a ball of energy and I have a lust for life. I'm the sort of person who makes the most of every day and I love to have fun. So for Steve, the cancer diagnosis was a bombshell. Before I had it confirmed, I remember him saying, 'Not you, it can't be you.' He just wasn't prepared for it.

He cried every morning in bed. One morning I thought, 'He's not going to be able to stop.' He was almost hysterical, sobbing so much I thought he was going to choke, and I was holding him and trying to be comforting. He's not a soft man at all, but he's sensitive and the thought that he might lose me was too much to bear.

It got to the point where I started thinking, 'I really don't know what I'm going to do here.' On the one hand I didn't want Steve to feel upset and I wanted to help him, but on the other hand I wanted to scream, 'Oh for Christ's sake. Come on!' because I needed him to rally and to try to be more positive.

Then one day when we were driving to Carluccio's in Esher for lunch, an email arrived on my phone from a lady who'd had exactly the same type of cancer as me ten years before. She told me my positive attitude was great and described how she'd got through her treatment and recovery. She was now in the clear and very healthy and happy. I read it out to Steve and when we got to the restaurant and sat down, he said, 'That's unbelievable. It's totally changed how I feel. I'm alright now.'

'Thank God!' I thought. It was such a brilliant email and it arrived just when we needed it. It was wonderful for both of us, but especially for Steve. Even though I'd told him we could beat it and I'd tried to buoy him up with my positivity, I don't think he actually believed it was possible until he read that email. I'll always be thankful to that woman because something just clicked for Steve that day and transformed his attitude. From then on he was amazing and he became my rock. He wouldn't so much as let me lift a coffee cup at the beginning, which in some ways was slightly annoying! But things settled down and he judged everything perfectly.

I was due to start chemo in May so the next thing I had to do was tell my family. I rang Maureen first. 'Are you sitting down?' I asked.

'Er, yes,' she replied. 'Why, what's wrong?'

'I've got some bad news I'm afraid, Maureen. I've got breast cancer.'

I heard a sharp intake of breath on the other end of the line and then sobbing.

'Sorry, I'll have to phone you back, Bernie,' she said, putting the phone down.

'Hmm, that went well!' I thought.

Next up was Linda. 'Oh shit!' was her response.

'But I'm not being negative, Linda,' I said before she had the chance to say anything else. 'I'm really positive about it. I'm going to have chemo for six months, then

I'm going to have a mastectomy and reconstruction and that's it. I don't want anybody to be down. Do you hear me?'

'Oh, God of course,' replied Linda. 'You'll be great. Look at me. I've beaten breast cancer and I'm fine now.'

She was fantastic and very positive.

I then called my brother Brian, who's such a softy. His immediate reaction was anger. 'Oh, fucking hell! Jesus Christ! What's going on in this family?' he said.

I gave him my little speech too. 'Look, I don't want any negative stuff, so you can stop that right now!' I said. 'We're going to fight this and everything's going to be fine.'

I asked Maureen, Linda and Brian to break the news to the others because I couldn't bear to call everyone.

Anne phoned as soon as she heard the news, even though we were still in the middle of the row we'd had over the reunion tour. But she didn't drag any of that up. She was very nice.

'I've just heard the news, Bernie,' she said. 'If there's anything you need, just let me know. If you need me to look after Erin, I can take time off work. We're all being positive for you and it'll turn out fine.'

I also received a lovely text from Denise, offering her help and support, and my eldest brother Tommy sent a message too. They were all fantastic.

The only one who didn't get in touch with me for a while was Coleen. I said to Steve one night, 'It's so odd that Coleen hasn't called. I know she's always busy, but there must be something else going on.' Then I spoke to Maureen, who told me that Coleen had been absolutely devastated by the news.

'She can't speak to you at the moment because she doesn't want to upset you and she can't talk without crying,' she explained.

It hit Coleen really hard. I think, like Steve, she was shocked because I'd always been such a strong person and so full of life and laughter. But that's no protection against cancer. Why shouldn't it happen to me?

Everyone gets over that initial shock, though. They have to. And Coleen did, too.

I was a bit apprehensive about chemotherapy, but I was also keen to get on with the treatment to start blitzing the cancer. I'd agreed to go on a trial for a drug called Pertuzumab, which I'd take along with three other drugs – Carboplatin, Herceptin and Docetaxel.

As anyone who's had chemo will tell you, the first session is an all-day affair. They have to put the drugs in slowly because they don't know how they're going to affect you. Some drugs take two hours to go in: drip, drip, drip. So Steve and I were fully prepared – we brought snacks and a laptop so we could watch DVDs.

I was given the first drug, Carboplatin, which was fine. The next one was Pertuzumab, the trial drug, which was also fine. Then the Herceptin went in – again, there were no problems. Finally, it was the turn of Docetaxel. The first drip went into my arm and I immediately felt like I couldn't breathe.

I turned to Steve, who was sitting in a chair reading. 'I can't breathe, Steve! And I feel hot, really hot,' I said, suddenly panicked.

'Oh my God, your face is bright red,' he said.

Just then, the nurse walked back into the room.

'I can't breathe,' I said, holding my throat. I literally couldn't take a breath. It was the worst feeling I've ever experienced and I remember thinking, 'This is what it must be like to die.'

She immediately switched off the drip and hit the alarm, then all hell broke loose. About six nurses and four doctors came rushing through the door. They gave me Piriton, an antihistamine, straight away.

I glanced up at Steve, who was standing in the doorway looking completely terrified. But as soon as the Piriton went in, I could breathe again.

I'd had a massive allergic reaction to the Docetaxel and, sadly, it meant I had to come off the trial, which I was devastated about because Pertuzumab was supposed to be a brilliant new drug. Even though I wasn't allergic to Pertuzumab itself, the trial was about that particular combination of drugs.

My biggest concern was that I hadn't had a full treatment, but the medical staff assured me I'd had plenty of drugs and not to let it worry me.

About two weeks after that first chemo session I went for a scan to find out how the tumours had responded to the treatment. I couldn't believe it when I was told they'd shrunk considerably – by more than 3cm. I think even my doctors were surprised by how successful it had been.

For my next chemo session I'd be taking a cocktail of Herceptin, Carboplatin and Taxol. To be honest, I'd been dreading chemo after what happened the first time, but the news that the tumours were shrinking gave me a real boost. Now I was looking forward to blasting them with more drugs!

'Keep thinking positive thoughts, Bernie,' I told myself. 'It's really working.'

10
A NEW LOOK

....

I never thought losing my hair would be a big deal for me, but it was.

I was in the shower one morning when I first noticed it was coming out. As I rinsed off the shampoo, a big clump of hair came away in my hand. 'Fuck!' I said, looking down at the blonde strands clinging to my wet fingers. It was a shocking moment, a wake-up call, a visual reminder that what was happening to me was real. 'Christ, I'm going to have no hair. What the hell will that look like?' I thought.

I got dressed hurriedly and went downstairs to the kitchen where Steve was cooking. 'Look at this, Steve,' I said, flicking my fingers through my hair and pulling it out with no effort at all.

'Well, you knew that was going to happen,' he said gently.

He was right, I was expecting it, but I still wasn't really prepared for it. It's very hard to accept if you're a woman – your hair is part of who you are. Losing it strikes right at the heart of your femininity.

The drug that makes it fall out is Carboplatin, so for my first two chemo sessions I opted to wear a cold cap to try to prevent it. That adds half an hour to your treatment though, and you have to keep it on the entire time, which is a bore, and it doesn't necessarily work. So after my second chemo session I thought, 'Sod it! I can't be bothered with this', and decided not to wear it for future treatments.

I started to get little bald patches all over my head, which looked pitiful. It made me look like an ill person. It was actually quite shocking for other people to see and it was traumatic for me, too. Maureen saw me once without a wig or a bandana and she told me afterwards that it had really upset her.

I decided I'd had enough of walking around with bald patches, looking sick. I actually felt really annoyed about it. I wanted to be in charge of how I looked. I didn't want cancer calling the shots. So one day, completely out of the blue, I said to Steve, 'Let's just shave it all off.'

I was doing some press at the time and I thought it might even help a few other women with cancer if they saw me bald. So I sat on the stool in the kitchen while Steve went to work with the clippers. We joked about it, which helped. 'If you make me bleed I'll kill ya!' I warned him. 'Don't worry, I do this on my own head all the time,' he said, laughing.

Afterwards he smoothed moisturiser over my head, so the skin was really soft. 'You look great,' he said, standing back to admire his work. 'It really suits you. You've actually got a lovely shaped head!'

A New Look

'Give us the mirror then,' I said, intrigued. When I looked at my reflection my initial reaction was, 'Wow! Not bad at all. Who knew I'd look OK bald?' I found I had a little strawberry birthmark on the back of my neck, which Mum never told me about, but she must have seen it when I was a baby. Amazing!

Steve took a photo of me with my newly shorn head on his mobile phone and went upstairs to show Erin. I wanted to lessen the shock for her. 'She says it looks cool,' he said when he came back down. 'Thank God,' I thought. I really didn't want Erin to be upset by it. However, she didn't like it when I went out in public bald and, to be honest, I wasn't that comfortable with it either because I did attract stares. Whenever she had friends coming over I'd ask, 'Wig, bandana or bald?' and, without hesitation, she'd always say 'Wig!'

Luckily, my friend Sally, who does my hair and make-up for press events and photo shoots, found me two fabulous wigs. One was real hair and the other was synthetic, and the synthetic one was actually easier to care for, so I ended up wearing it most of the time. It was long to begin with, but Sally came over to the house one day and while we were outside in the garden having a glass of wine, she cut and styled it on me, so it looked similar to my own hair before it had fallen out. I was so chuffed with it and Steve couldn't get over how real it looked. I can't tell you how much better it made me feel – I felt like Bernie again.

A couple of weeks later, I went to Maureen's hen party at her friend's house in Blackpool wearing my synthetic wig. A couple of the girls who didn't know me came over and said, 'God you look great, how's the chemo going? We thought your hair fell out.'

'It did!' I said. 'This is a wig.' They couldn't believe it.

And later when the lads arrived – they'd been at the pub – Maureen's partner Richie came over to chat to me. We've known each other for years and we've always got on brilliantly.

'You look absolutely stunning, but I thought you were going to get a wig,' he said.

'This is a wig!' I repeated.

'Fuck off!' he said. 'Oh my God, it's amazing.'

Then he almost made me cry because he added, 'We're all so proud of you, Bernie. So proud of you.'

We had such a laugh that night. I love a party and it was wonderful to cut loose and have fun. We played bingo, the food was great and there was a guitarist there too, so of course Maureen made me sing. As I've already said, she's my biggest fan! The first song I did was 'I Can't Make You Love Me' by Bonnie Raitt, which is beautiful. Funnily enough, this time the mood was different because everyone was crying. And obviously I knew why. When I finished I said, 'You morbid bunch of bastards. I know why you're crying. You can all get stuffed!' and we all fell about laughing. But it was poignant because I knew it was because they cared and were thinking about what I was going through.

Later on, before the men turned up, someone had the idea that we should all jump in the hot tub. I was wearing a very expensive Karen Millen dress. 'Hmmm,' I thought. 'I do want to go in the hot tub, but I'm not ruining this dress,' so I took it off, hung it up, and went in wearing just my knickers. Well, there was murder because Linda was horrified, which made me laugh because she's the so-called 'Naughty Nolan', the one who'd done all these sexy shoots years ago. But she was disgusted with me!

'Oh Bernie, I can't believe you're doing that,' she said, eyes wide with shock. 'Someone could take a picture and it might end up in the papers.'

'Chill out!' I said, sinking up to my neck in the warm water and taking a slug of wine. My niece Amy was sitting next to me giggling. 'These women are my mates. It's just a pair of breasts! Who cares? I won't have one of them soon!'

Then the girl who was throwing the party brought me a T-shirt so I put it on, but I couldn't understand Linda's prim and proper attitude. I was just sitting in a hot tub with loads of other women. It was no big deal.

I had a brilliant time that night, but there were low moments that summer, too. After that first awful chemo session I did really well on the drugs, thank goodness, but it was still a big deal having the treatment every six weeks. The tiredness could be overwhelming, but I refused to just sit around and wait for the symptoms to hit me. Sometimes we'd be out shopping in town and I'd have to ask Steve to take me home straight away. It was the kind of tiredness you couldn't fight.

And after the second round of chemo I started getting mouth ulcers, which were a side effect of the drugs. At one point I had twenty-five of them and they were incredibly painful and debilitating. I couldn't eat, I couldn't drink, I couldn't sleep. My mouth used to bleed and stick together at night, so I had to prise my lips open in the morning. I'm not one to moan, but this was hard. It was so bad they had to take me off the drugs and I missed a whole month of chemo. It was the only time during my whole six months of treatment that I cried my eyes out.

But the way I look at it is, you can make it worse or you can make it better, and I definitely always made it better by trying to find something positive. I'd think, 'OK, so chemo might be hard sometimes and I'm bald and I've got mouth ulcers, but it's going to keep me alive, so who gives a damn?' I don't know if I always had that in me or if it was something that happened as a reaction to getting cancer, but it helped. And I'd constantly remind myself of everything good in my life – a fantastic husband, a great kid, a wonderful job. The power of positive thinking is amazing. Even if I'd started out trying to convince myself things would be OK, eventually I started to believe it.

There was one day in particular that really brought home to me how powerful your mind can be. I'd promised to take Erin to the Capital FM Summertime Ball at the O2 in London and she'd been so looking forward to it. My chemo had been going well, but on the morning of the concert I woke up feeling really bad. I had terrible backache and just felt weird. I didn't say anything to Erin because she was so excited. Steve wasn't that keen to spend the entire day with thousands of screaming girls and I really wanted to be the one to go with her. He said he'd drive us there, so the three of us piled into the car. All the way there I kept saying to Steve, 'God, my back is agony.'

'I'll take her,' he said. 'You drive the car home and we'll get the train back.'

But I was determined to do it because there was a little part of me that worried I might not be here next year to take her. It's one of the few times I've ever thought that way, but it did go through my head. Something was telling me it was important to take her, so I did and we had one of the best mother and daughter days out we've ever had. I took paracetamol every few hours to numb the pain and mustered up the strength to climb up and down the stairs to get us drinks and burgers. And I was able to carry on for six or seven hours, watching all these bands and singers Erin loved – Rihanna, Pixie Lott, JLS and Justin Bieber. And it was brilliant to see her enjoying herself, singing and dancing along to the music. I even managed to stand up and sing with her, which her dad would never have done! It's a day that will always stick out in my mind. It had started out as one of the worst days I'd experienced on chemo, but turned into one of my best days ever. And I'm convinced that if I'd have stayed at home and sat on the sofa, I would have been in agony all day. So there is something to be said for getting up and getting on with things if you can.

This will probably sound ridiculous, given that I was in the middle of chemo, but that summer was one of the best for us as a family. I was so glad I'd decided to give up work. I did the school run with Erin every day and Steve did all the cooking. We were a proper family unit and it helped give me the strength and energy to fight my illness. We laughed a lot, we had parties and, instead of going abroad for a summer holiday, we spent a fortnight travelling around England, visiting friends and family we don't get to see enough. It culminated in Blackpool with the Nolan clan and Erin had a ball. We did all the stuff I'd done as a kid – the Pleasure Beach, Blackpool Tower, Stanley Park and the zoo. We also visited friends in Newcastle and Birmingham, and saw Steve's family and his best mate in Stockton.

Before I'd been diagnosed with breast cancer, we'd planned to go to Maureen and Richie's wedding in Spain that August. But once I'd started my treatment, I didn't know if I'd feel up to it or if I'd actually be allowed to leave the country while I was still having chemo. But as the date drew nearer, I was desperate not to miss it and I felt fine. I checked with my oncologist Dr Houston and he gave me permission to go. He also gave me a letter that detailed my condition so that if I was taken unwell in Spain, I could just hand it over to the doctors. The only thing he expressly told me not to do was sunbathe, as my skin was sensitive because of the chemotherapy drugs. I was even allowed to have a glass of champagne. 'Good,' I thought. 'I need to let off some steam!'

Although I was looking forward to the wedding, it was scary too, because I was one of Maureen's bridesmaids and I didn't want to walk down that aisle looking like I had a wig on or looking ill. In fact, I worried about it for a whole week before we went, which is very unlike me.

Maureen and Richie own an apartment in Almeria, so we rented one in the same block, which a few of the other guests also decided to do so we could all be together. It has a lovely pool and the weather was gorgeous when we arrived. Steve, Erin and I were more than ready for a few days of chilling out in the sun. Boy, did we need it!

And I really needn't have worried – everyone was great and they looked after me really well. In the mornings when I came down to the pool, they'd all be running around trying to fetch me a chair so I could sit in the shade.

We had a few days to kill before the wedding and there were fun things planned every evening. All the girls would get dressed up in their finery to go dancing or out for dinner, which I felt slightly intimidated by, and I had to make sure I left enough time to get my wig on properly and apply my false eyelashes!

During the day, I wore a bandana because it was too hot to put on a wig. One day, someone took a picture of Maureen, Linda and me by the pool and at the time I thought I looked awful. But I've looked at it since and I look absolutely fine – and the bandana is lovely.

The wedding day itself was very exciting. Linda, Coleen and I were bridesmaids, Erin and Ciara were flower girls and Maureen's son Danny gave her away. They'd planned to have an open-air ceremony at a lovely hotel called La Envia just down the road from our apartments. There were dozens of pretty white chairs lined up in the garden, but when we got up that morning it was raining – in Spain, in August! None of us could believe it. When we were having our make-up done, sipping champagne and having a laugh, Linda whispered to me, 'Oh my God, it's raining. Don't let Maureen look out the window!'

Rick, the best man, kept calling us, saying, 'What shall I do? We need to decide now whether to go inside.' In the end, he made the decision to stay outside, but when it came time for the wedding, the rain miraculously stopped, the sun came out and it was dazzling.

I wore a lavender bridesmaid's gown and my real hair wig, which had been styled to resemble the hairstyle I'd had when we did the reunion tour, and I felt fabulous. I was so relieved I looked the part. No one would have known I was ill.

It was magical when Maureen walked down the aisle, which was lined with beautiful white flowers. She looked simply stunning.

That night I booked Steve, Erin and me into the hotel so we wouldn't have to walk back up the hill to the apartments. It cost a fortune, but it was totally worth it. I got very drunk and we danced until dawn. It was brilliant!

In September I had my last chemotherapy session and that night Steve and I cracked open a bottle of champagne to celebrate. I had this wonderful feeling of euphoria – I'd got through it and it was over! We also found out that the type of breast cancer I had wasn't genetic, which meant Erin wasn't at any more risk of getting the disease than anyone else. Thank God! I cried with relief and happiness. It was a huge boost. Linda's breast cancer hadn't been genetic either, so I guess we'd just been incredibly unlucky that three of us in one family had developed it.

Of course, I still had to have the mastectomy and

reconstruction, which was scheduled for 8 October. I was anxious about that because it was major surgery and I'd be under anaesthetic for eight hours, but I told myself I'd cross that bridge when I got to it.

I also attended the TV Choice Awards at the Dorchester Hotel in London in September. It was my first red carpet appearance since I'd lost my hair. That day I'd been at a photo shoot for *Best* magazine, so my make-up was gorgeous and they'd styled my real hair wig, which also looked amazing. But when I put on my beautiful dress and looked in the mirror, I thought, 'Hmm, this is wrong, it just doesn't feel right.' So I took off the wig and looked again. 'Yep, that's much better!' Bald was going to be my look for the night. How could I miss the opportunity to show solidarity with other women fighting breast cancer? Most people don't have a make-up artist at their fingertips or the money to splash out on a real hair wig. This was a great chance to stick two fingers up at cancer and say: 'So what? I'm bald!' And it was a good decision. The paparazzi went nuts when I turned up and my picture was in all the papers the next morning. I got an amazing reaction afterwards. People came up to me in the street and said things like, 'You're doing a great job, Bernie. Keep fighting.' Or they told me how much my story had helped someone in their family. I received so many letters and emails of thanks, which was incredibly touching and unexpected.

I never wanted cancer to define me and I still don't because there's so much more to me than that, but I've accepted it is part of my journey now. And I've learnt so much about myself and other people because of it. When you're fighting cancer, all the important things in life suddenly come into sharp focus and everything else just melts away. All that mattered to me were the people I loved and holding on to this wonderful life of mine.

11
BEING BERNIE AGAIN

....

The night before my operation, all I remember thinking was, 'I want my mum.' I still can't believe she's gone and since becoming so ill, I've missed her more every day. When you're sick and frightened only your mum will do, right? And I was scared, to the point where I really had to steel myself for the next day. I didn't cry, but I felt like I wanted to. Luckily, we managed to sleep OK that night, as we had to be at the Royal Surrey for 6 a.m.

After I'd arrived at the hospital and got changed into my hospital gown, a doctor came round to check my weight and blood pressure and so on. 'Have you got a cough?' he asked.

I did have a cold and cough, which had been playing on my mind because I was worried they wouldn't go ahead with the op.

'Yeah, but it's not a bad one,' I said, dismissing it with a wave of my hand.

I really wanted to have the surgery that day because I'd built myself up for it. I couldn't face going through another 'night before' scenario. The doctor left the room and when he came back a few minutes later he said, 'It's OK, you're fine. They're going to do it.'

Within half an hour I was on a trolley, ready to be wheeled down to theatre. Steve and I kissed and hugged. 'You'll be great. I'll be there when you come out and I'll be there when you wake up,' he said. He was on the verge of tears, but he held it together for me.

I was anxious, not just because it was a major op and I was having my breast removed, but I didn't know what else they'd find. They might find cancer in my nipple, so I wouldn't be able to keep it and they could find that the disease had spread to my lymph nodes.

Steve walked alongside the trolley as we made our way through the hospital corridors, holding my hand for as long as he could, until we got to the door and just our fingertips were touching. 'I love you,' he said.

'I love you, too.'

I was taken into a kind of holding room where I had a pre-med and I'll never forget the moment I turned my head to look out of the window. It was still very early and the morning light was beautiful. Whatever they'd given me helped me to feel calm. Outside someone had painted a big sunflower on the wall opposite my window and when I saw it, I felt completely at peace. 'I'm going to be OK,' I thought, and I didn't feel scared any more.

Mr Kissin came into the room and proceeded to draw all over me, marking where he was going to cut. 'Oh, this is attractive,' I joked, and we both laughed. And that was the last thing I remembered before waking up in the recovery room after surgery.

'Oh, you're awake!' a nurse said, coming over to check

on me. 'Yeah, I'm awake,' I replied, thinking how odd it was that I couldn't feel any pain. I was wheeled back to the ward, still feeling pretty drugged up, and I remember seeing a lonely figure sitting in a chair. 'God love him,' I thought, before I realised it was Steve!

'Hi, how are ya?' I said before he had the chance to ask how I was!

'God, I'm fine!' he said, clearly relieved to see me and that I was 'being Bernie'. He told me later, though, that he cried his eyes out when I was taken into surgery. The nurses advised him to go home because the op was so long, but when he got home he couldn't sit still. 'I just needed to be close to you. I needed to be in the same building,' he told me. So he sat outside the ward all day in a plastic chair, waiting for me to return.

The day after the op, I woke up and thought, 'I might as well look at it now, just face it.' I already knew I'd been able to keep my nipple, which I was hugely relieved about. Mark Kissin also sits you up when you're under, so he can measure your boobs, and he said, 'I made it to match the other one, so there's a little bit of sag in it.'

'God, how embarrassing!' I thought. So I asked one of the nurses to help me and I had a peek at my new breast. And, although I had stitches and it was still terribly swollen, I could see beyond that and I could tell that Mr Kissin had done an amazing job. I'd imagined it'd be much worse. The stuff you make up in your head is often worse than the reality. When Steve arrived at the hospital that morning I asked if he wanted to see it and he hesitated. 'I don't know. Maybe not yet,' he said.

'Don't worry, I totally get it,' I reassured him. I think he left that day feeling really bad, which is silly, because we all need to do things at our own pace.

I had to stay in hospital for a week after the op and there were some horrendous days, if I'm honest. That first morning I was told I had to stay lying flat on my back. 'OK,' I thought, 'I can do that,' so I watched telly and I texted my family and friends to say I was fine and that I was lying in bed eating Maltesers. No one could believe it, but I actually felt fine. It probably had something to do with relief, euphoria and painkillers all rolled into one! Every now and then the nurses would come in and change the bags that the fluid from my back and breast was draining into.

However, the lying flat part started to really bother me and I had to have a hot blanket over me too, which looked a bit like bubble wrap. Hospitals are so hot anyway and during the night this blanket would stick to my face, and I'd wake up with it over my face, which was awful because I was lying flat. I felt so claustrophobic. In fact, one night I had a panic attack, but I couldn't move because I still had to be lifted. 'I need to sit up! I can't breathe!' I called out to one of the nurses, who rushed over and sat me up. 'You're alright,' she said soothingly.

I began to hate lying on my back and I despised the hot blanket, but having to use a bedpan was probably the worst thing about my whole time in hospital. Mr Kissin doesn't believe in catheters so it was bedpans all the way. I found it so humiliating. Invariably it would spill over and go all over the bed. I absolutely dreaded it.

After a few days, things got better – I was able to sit up and they started bringing food, which was pretty vile to be honest, but I didn't have much of an appetite. I was in quite good spirits though. Linda was staying at ours to look after Erin and do the school run while Steve went back and forward to the hospital. Then Maureen surprised me with a visit, which was lovely. She'd come all the way from Blackpool.

Just before I was due to be discharged I was finally ready for the commode. It was during the night and one of the nurses sat me on it and I fainted forward. All I remember is her screaming the other nurse's name, 'Mary! Mary!' The next thing I remember was waking up in bed, lying flat on my back with these two gorgeous nurses holding my wrists and hands. 'Hi Bernie. You OK?' one of them asked. 'You just fainted. It's nothing serious; you're just not used to standing up.'

I was brought a cup of tea and the nurses stayed with me, chatting. They don't get enough praise for what they do. After I left I sent them a hamper of sweets and cakes because I'd noticed they were always eating!

After that I started to get stronger and could get up on my own and go to the toilet in my room. I never thought I'd say this in my life, but it was absolutely wonderful just being able to walk to the toilet! No bedpan, no commode – fabulous!

I remember the first day I was able to get up, I applied a bit of mascara and when Steve came to visit later he said, 'Look at you, you look great!' It was good for him to see me looking more like my old self.

During the surgery, Mr Kissin had taken out thirteen

lymph nodes, which thankfully all turned out to be free of cancer. It was a major boost.

The last hurdle I had to face before going home was getting some of the drains taken out. I was a bit scared, simply because I didn't know what to expect, but it was nothing. They told me to breathe in and, as I did, they pulled out the drain. I didn't feel a thing.

I felt so excited the day I was going home. Maureen and Linda came to the hospital to help me get my things together. When I got back to the house they helped me get comfortable on the sofa, which was pretty much my home for the next ten days. Just as I'd settled in, though, my little dog Dexter came rushing over and pulled the bag with my drains in it! I could feel a tug on my back and let out a big yelp. He was just happy to see me, but it could have been disastrous!

I'd got out of hospital on 15 October and my fiftieth birthday was two days later – this wasn't exactly how I'd imagined it to be! When I woke up that morning it was a beautiful sunny autumn day and when Steve asked me what I wanted to do, I said I wanted to be outside in the sunshine, so we decided to go to a pub in Walton-on-Thames and have lunch. Maureen and Linda were there, my brother Brian and his wife Annie, and my best mate Rick Coates. Maureen's husband Richie turned up to surprise me later that evening and Steve cooked us a fabulous meal and we had birthday cake afterwards. It was perfect. I felt very lucky and happy to be with the people I loved, full of hope and feeling good. And it was great to see Steve relaxing and having a beer for the first time in ages.

I still had a couple of drains in, which wasn't pleasant, and Erin hated them. But that day Linda had this big beautiful leather handbag with her. 'Put your drains in here, Bernie,' she said. Classy, eh? I thought it was a brilliant idea – much more chic and discreet than a carrier bag! One thing I really believe in is that if you make yourself look better, you'll feel better, too. Throughout my chemo and recovery from surgery I always made an effort with my appearance. Every morning I applied make-up, coloured in my brows with a pencil and applied false eyelashes – I can apply falsies almost blind now! And I always wore a colourful bandana, a hat or one of my wigs. Even if I felt like shit, I didn't want to look like shit! And it gave me a boost when other people said how well I was looking. I didn't want anyone to see me looking really sick. Maureen saw me just after my op with no wig or make-up and she was heartbroken. It's tough to see a loved one like that.

With each day that went by, my breast began to look better and better. When Steve first saw it, he said straight away, 'Oh my God, it's amazing!' He couldn't get over how good it looked. In fact, everyone who's seen it has had the same reaction. It looks just the same as my other boob and the scar is tiny and straight. I wanted to shout from the rooftops about my new boob and show it to everyone!

About four weeks after the surgery I had the remaining drains removed, which was a huge relief, although I still had to go back to the hospital every so often to have my back drained. On the run-up to Christmas, I started to feel like myself again. My hair had grown back into a little crewcut, although it was now curly and ash grey, so I dyed it immediately! My back was still sore – I think it's going to be tender in parts forever. After the op, Mark explained that he'd had to go quite deep into my back to get enough muscle for the reconstruction. He reckoned my muscles were probably weaker because I'd been a smoker – even though I'd given up fifteen years before. Another reason not to smoke!

But apart from my back still being a little sore and stiff, I felt wonderful. And the best thing of all was finding out just before Christmas that my scans were clear – I was told they'd got all the cancer. The chemo and mastectomy had been incredibly successful and I was in remission. Now I just had to keep going until that magic five-year 'all clear' milestone. It was brilliant news. I could finally relax and look forward to spending Christmas with Steve and Erin. There had obviously been bleak moments during my treatment when the days seemed to drag on forever, but in just eight months I'd gone from diagnosis to remission. It was extraordinary.

I absolutely adore Christmas – it's my favourite time of year by far, probably because it was such a big deal in the Nolan house when we were kids. Every year I go nuts decorating our house with fairy lights, candles and the tallest real tree I can squeeze into our living room. I even spray snow on the windowpanes! I'm sure Steve and Erin think I'm nuts!

When I was still living at home I remember being devastated the first year Anne told us she wouldn't be coming over for Christmas. 'What do you mean?' I asked, horrified.

'Um, I've got a husband and daughters now and we'd like to spend Christmas in our own home,' she replied, completely reasonably. But I couldn't get over it. I was so upset, even though she came round after dinner for the present opening!

After we moved to Ilford, we still tried to get the family together for Christmas. My brothers would come down from Blackpool with their girlfriends or wives. And, after I moved out, I'd still come home, usually with a boyfriend – and occasionally his family – in tow! But my mum loved it. 'The more the merrier,' she'd say. It was always a party.

After Mum and Dad died, everyone gradually started having Christmases with their own families. But I still like to see as many of my family as possible over Christmas to keep that tradition alive for Mum and Dad.

But Christmas 2010 was shaping up to be the most special one of all. Linda, Brian and Annie, and Maureen and Richie were all coming to stay. I was amazed that Richie was being prised out of Blackpool, but I think they were all coming because I'd been ill. In the past Steve, Erin and I had always travelled up North to see the family over the holidays.

I really went to town, putting candles and welcome gifts in their rooms and little chocolates on their pillows. I'd set the dinner table beautifully with little presents and hired seat covers with big satin bows. We had five live lobsters in the fridge on Christmas Eve, which we called the Jackson Five! Steve is a brilliant cook and he'd planned a fabulous menu with a different wine for each course. We had fresh lobster cocktail with mango to start, a vodka sorbet as an in-between course, traditional roast turkey with all the trimmings, including homemade chestnut stuffing and cranberry sauce, then Christmas pudding or homemade tarte tatin for pudding. We ended with cheese and biscuits, and champagne for toasts.

Steve made a lovely speech, reflecting on what we'd been through that year. 'Look at her, she's here with her little crewcut,' he said, raising his champagne flute. 'Her hair is growing back, she's got two gorgeous breasts, and she's still my beautiful Bernie. And we've got it all to look forward to.' It was very moving and I felt so fortunate to be sitting there with my family around me. Then, being the Nolans, we all sang carols around the table. It was such a happy day.

On Boxing Day lots of our friends came over for a quiz night and brought their leftovers, then Steve, Erin and I spent New Year's Eve at home on our own, which was fitting. The three of us had battled through the toughest year of our lives together – a strong little unit. We had a lot to be thankful for and a lot to celebrate in the coming year.

In January, I was straight into rehearsals for my first job since I'd been diagnosed – playing Cora in *Calendar Girls*, which would require me being topless on stage! For those of you who don't know it, it's based on the true story of a group of Women's Institute ladies who group together to shoot a charity calendar with a difference, following the death of one of their husbands from cancer. In the shots they're doing everyday things completely naked, with strategically placed objects such as cupcakes and teapots protecting their modesty! Sunflowers are a prominent theme in the production because the husband who inspired the story grew them throughout his cancer treatment and gave them to his friends and family, hoping that when they bloomed, he would have beaten the disease. Strangely, it had been a sunflower painted on the wall outside my hospital room that had helped me find peace on the morning of my surgery.

For me, it was an inspiring role to come back with. Originally, I'd been asked to do it in 2010, but then I was diagnosed with breast cancer and had to call the producer, David Pugh, and tell him I'd have to pull out. 'Well, keep January and February 2011 free,' he said. 'We've got another tour starting then and you're doing that one, OK?'

'Yep, you're on! Thanks,' I replied, unable to believe how lucky I was to work with such kind people.

I was playing the part of the piano player, so I would have my back to the audience, where I had a lot of scarring, so it was quite a big thing to do. But I wanted to show other women that you can do anything if you put your mind to it and that scarring is nothing to be ashamed of.

Of course the audience doesn't see you completely starkers because there are props cleverly covering your bits, but everyone on stage does. If anybody was shy they had to get over it!

We got the naked bit out of the way on the first

rehearsal and of course all the girls saw my false boob. I thought I'd get in there first to save any embarrassment. 'I just wanted to let you all know that I've only got one real boob, so that one is going to look crap,' I joked, showing them my boobs. Everyone fell about laughing and they all thought the reconstruction was amazing.

'Let me show you the scars on my back now,' I said, turning round and lifting up my T-shirt. It actually felt good to get it all out in the open.

My fellow cast members were a great bunch of girls and included Lynda Bellingham, Ruth Madoc, Lisa Riley, Jennifer Ellison, who I'd done *Brookside* with, and Trudie Goodwin, who I'd worked with on *The Bill*. And Joe McGann was playing the husband who'd inspired the story.

Our opening night was in Dublin on 8 February and it was pretty nerve-wracking, if I'm honest. The cast had got used to seeing each other naked in rehearsals, so that part was fine. And for the scene where we drop our robes they clear the backstage area too. I think I was more nervous because I didn't know how the audience would react to the scarring on my back, plus it was my first role in nearly a year.

When it was my turn to get naked, I had to undo my robe and let it drape down over the piano stool, so the audience could see the whole of my back and my butt cheeks – and my scar of course. As soon as the robe dropped a huge cheer went up and I got a massive round of applause. It actually made me cry. It was so touching that people were rooting for me. And after that first night

I didn't worry about it any more, I just did it. Steve was in the audience for the first show and he was really proud of me, too.

I'm so glad I said yes to *Calendar Girls*. It was liberating and empowering, and it gave me confidence. Each night, at the end of the play, we all lifted up part of the set and sunflowers came up on stage, which was a beautiful and poignant moment, even more so for me because I'd seen that sunflower before my operation. It was amazing. It felt as if I'd come full circle.

Things were going well at home too. I was so grateful for Steve and Erin. Linda's husband Brian died while she was having chemotherapy, and I'm not sure I would have been as brave as she was if I hadn't had Steve and Erin to fall back on. Erin supported me just by being herself – being strong and sensible when things were tough. She's always been wise beyond her years.

And I can't imagine anybody being as wonderful as Steve. Of course we argue like any couple – we're both very independent and headstrong – but he's a good person and we love each other. I know how lucky I am to have fallen in love with somebody like him.

It's tough for any man to see his partner go through breast cancer. As well as the fear and the emotional fallout, Steve also had to deal with the physical changes in my body. Sexually speaking, it can be a minefield, but if you're close enough as a couple, you get through it. I'm sure with most guys there's a bit of 'Should I just touch the real one?' Or 'Will she be offended if I avoid the fake one?' Steve and I could always laugh about things, which really helped.

Naturally, when you're going through gruelling treatment and during your recovery, your sex life becomes non-existent. Sex was the furthest thing from my mind – it seemed so trivial. I was fighting for my life; a bonk wasn't going to help! But, again, it's hard for your partner because he's healthy and still has natural urges.

Steve and I had always been a very physical couple – it wasn't everything, but it was a big part of our relationship. Every cloud has a silver lining though, and what not having sex did was to make us realise how much deeper our relationship went. We found out so much more about each other and about ourselves. Our relationship developed into something more beautiful and meaningful. We just felt closer because of what we were going through.

In the past we might have solved a row by coming together physically – you know, make-up sex! But now we couldn't do that, so we had to talk things through properly and have a hug and kiss instead. We had always known our relationship was good, but we didn't know how good until cancer came into our lives and tested it.

We didn't make love for about six months after my surgery. Once all the drips and drains had come out and my scars had healed, I then had to deal with the onset of the menopause, which the chemo drugs had brought on. Luckily, my symptoms weren't severe – I didn't get hot flushes or mood swings, but I didn't feel much like sex. Luckily neither did Steve. Occasionally, one of us would say, 'My God, we haven't had sex for ages!' And the other would reply, 'I know . . . I'm not bothered, are you?' We didn't need it to keep us together, thank God.

But when we did get round to it, things happened naturally. What I'd say to women going through the same thing is don't put pressure on yourself – work up to it slowly. Without wishing to sound crude, there's plenty of other stuff you can do apart from penetrative sex. People tend to shy away from discussing the impact something like breast cancer has on your sex life, but it's important to get it out in the open.

After finishing *Calendar Girls* in April, I decided to take the whole summer off. Steve, Erin and I escaped to Florida for a long, long holiday. Erin adores the place – we used to go when she was little and we've got tons of videos and photos of all the lovely times we've spent there. We were all very, very excited, especially Erin, because we'd booked a Disney hotel called the Swan. We splashed out big time to go fully inclusive and the hotel provided little ferries to and from the Disney resorts. It felt really special and relaxing. It was Erin's birthday on 26 April, so I booked a 'Whodunnit' dinner where actors joined us between courses, playing out a crime drama and we had to guess who the culprit was. It was great fun and we guessed right. Erin was a bit annoyed because her dad and I won a bottle of champagne and she got a really cheap little kid's bag!

Steve and Erin went on every rollercoaster – twice! And I managed to go on nearly all of them – not bad considering I'd recently had a mastectomy. It was a truly magical holiday and one I'll never forget.

I also organised my long-overdue fiftieth birthday party for May 2011. I wanted a major bash and invited 200 friends and relatives – I had a lot to celebrate after all! On the Friday before the party, everyone began arriving. I'd arranged a drink and a meal for twenty of us in Weybridge that night. We all met at the Queen's Head on the High Street for a drink, then walked to the tapas bar on Baker Street and had a wonderful meal, lots of lovely wine and so much fun! I went to bed that night fairly drunk, but very happy.

The next day, Steve and I drove to the Oatlands Park Hotel, a beautiful place with gorgeous grounds and a lake at the end of a tree-lined garden. Our suite had a four-poster bed and a lovely view overlooking the grounds. It was so special. I was beyond thrilled!

Steve and me were having tea and sandwiches in the reception area when my guests started to arrive. Everyone was kissing, hugging and laughing. I was already having a ball and the party hadn't even started!

My make-up girl Sally arrived to glam me up for the night – she'd been doing my hair and make-up since the promo for The Nolans' reunion tour and had sorted me out with those wonderful wigs when I lost my hair through chemo. My hair had grown back, but it was very short and I still had no eyelashes or eyebrows, so Sally worked wonders with make-up pencils and false eyelashes to make me look lovely. She's a true artiste and a genuinely wonderful human being. After putting on some glam diamanté earrings and slipping into my full-length cream satin Karen Millen dress, Steve and I hit the hotel bar, where we'd arranged to meet everyone.

Steve did an amazing job with the music, which he'd

arranged on his computer – from welcome music and drinks music to sit-down-and-eat music and dance music! He'd thought of everything. He also arranged a sixteen-piece live band for a sort of cabaret show and the running order and keys were all sorted beforehand so there was no karaoke-type wait while they worked out what they wanted to sing and in what key. Amazing! Our good friend Duncan Waugh, a music director, really helped us out with that.

My favourite part of the whole night was when Erin sang a solo. She'd already told me she wasn't going to sing, so I was totally clueless about it. She sang 'When Somebody Loved Me' from *Toy Story 2* and Steve accompanied her on keyboards. I sobbed my heart out at the end and hugged her tight. I was so deeply touched.

My brother Brian sang and so did Anne, Maureen, Linda and Coleen. My mate Drew sang 'Lately' unbelievably well, my longtime friend Bobby Ball sang and so did my friend Andi from Newcastle, who has a voice just like Gladys Knight. Steve sang three or four songs – he really outdid himself! Peter Cox performed, too, and his version of 'Your Sex Is On Fire' by The Kings of Leon was spectacular. I couldn't believe he'd sung at *my* party! He was so nice and I think all the girls were a little infatuated with him. Can't think why! It was truly special. We danced until 2 a.m. and then sat in the bar until 4 a.m. It was beautiful and I'll never forget it or the effort everyone made to be there.

It was a wonderful summer – I felt well again and filled with optimism. And I'm glad Steve, Erin and I got the opportunity to spend some proper time together as a family because I had a lot of work lined up for the end of the year and throughout 2012.

I'd signed up for panto in Stevenage, playing Malevolent in *Beauty and the Beast*. It was my first job since *Calendar Girls* and I was overjoyed to be performing again. And when that wrapped up towards the end of January, I went straight into three weeks of rehearsals for a production of *Chicago*, which opened on 10 February in Bradford. I was playing the part of Mama Morton – a wonderful strong lesbian character. Ali Bastian was Roxie Hart, Stefan Booth was playing Billy Flynn and Tupele Dorgu was Velma Kelly. It was a ten-month nationwide tour with a few shows in glamorous Monte Carlo along the way, and my old friend David Ian was the producer. I was hugely excited to be part of it because *Chicago* is such a prestigious show.

It was a pretty hectic few months because I didn't have a break between panto and *Chicago*, but I've always loved being busy and I just felt really grateful that I was well enough to work.

Looking back, 2011 had been a great year, even though I was still recovering from surgery. I felt so blessed to be in remission and I honestly didn't dwell on the thought the cancer could return – as you know by now, my cup is always half full. But if somebody asked me if I was 'cured' or if I'd been given the 'all clear', I would always say, 'No, I'm in remission.' Every day I got more used to my new breast and my back became less sore. I felt I had everything to look forward to and I was back on stage, doing what I loved most.

12
APRIL ALWAYS BRINGS BAD NEWS

....

One evening in April 2012, I was in the bedroom getting ready to go out for dinner with Steve. I just had my bra on and was sitting at the dressingtable doing my make-up, and as I lifted my arm to brush my hair I noticed a lump on the left side of my chest. 'God, that doesn't look right,' I thought. So I moved my other arm in the same way, but couldn't see anything similar on the right side.

Just then, Steve walked into the room, so I called him over to have a look. 'Oh, it's probably just the muscle. Don't worry,' he said reassuringly. I was due to go for a mammogram on my natural breast in a fortnight's time, so I decided to ask about the lump then.

This time the mammogram was at the Royal Surrey, where I'd had my cancer treatment. At my appointment I flagged up the lump to the breast care nurse straight away. 'I've spotted a lump here,' I said, moving my fingers over it. 'Can you check it out?'

'Yes, I can feel it,' she said. 'I'll get our radiographer to have a look.'

Luckily, the radiographer was free and did a scan

there and then. 'You're right, there is a lump and I think we'll need to do a biopsy on it,' she said. 'We can do it now.'

As soon as I heard the word 'biopsy' my heart sank to the pit of my stomach, but I was already at the hospital and I'm all about early detection, so I braced myself and said, 'You'd better do it,' adding quickly that I hated biopsies.

'Don't worry, I'll hold your hand,' said the nurse, so I took her hand and held it tightly as the needle went in. When it was over I was told they wouldn't be able to tell if the lump was cancerous until I got the results of the biopsy and to expect to hear from them in a week's time. I knew the drill. It felt like *Groundhog Day*.

Steve was sitting outside in the waiting-room and when I saw him I raised my eyes up to heaven, so he knew immediately that things hadn't gone to plan. 'What is it?' he asked, getting up from his chair.

'I've had a biopsy on the lump,' I said.

'Oh God,' was all Steve could say.

We walked through the hospital corridors in silence and as we got outside he said, 'It'll be fine, Bernie. It can't happen again, that would be ridiculous.'

'OK, let's go and eat,' I said. All sorts of different scenarios were rushing through my mind, but I was determined to stay strong for Steve and Erin.

The mammogram was on a Friday and I was due back at work in *Chicago* the following Monday. The show was in Eastbourne that week and it was the Easter holidays, so I took Steve and Erin with me. When I'm on tour they come with me whenever they can – if Erin's off school and Steve's not working.

We had a nice time – the flat was lovely and the three of us went for a walk up to Beachy Head one day, which is beautiful. And there was a great pub nearby where the cast would go after the show. I've got pictures of us all singing in there one night. It was good fun.

Then on the Friday morning about 8 a.m., Steve and I were still in bed when my mobile rang. It was one of my breast cancer nurses, Jill. As soon as I heard her voice, I knew it wasn't going to be good news.

'I'm sorry to say that your cancer is back, Bernie,' she said. 'We did find cancer in the lump.'

When I put the phone down, I turned to Steve. 'It's back,' I said.

This time I was more pissed off than anything else. I felt a combination of boiling rage and disbelief. 'Christ!' I thought. 'Surely I've been through enough – dead babies, breast cancer, a mastectomy, my parents dying?'

'What did she say?' said Steve, sitting up.

'Well, Mr Kissin wants to see me on Sunday to talk about the next step.'

We packed up our things that day and headed back to London. We didn't tell Erin or anybody else.

Steve came with me to my appointment on the Sunday where Mark Kissin explained that he was going to remove the lump and give me radiotherapy. 'OK, that doesn't sound too bad,' I thought.

I was also pleased because I'd still be able to go to Monte Carlo with *Chicago* the following Wednesday, provided I could fit in some scans before I went – a CT scan, a PET-CT scan, a bone scan and a heart scan. Steve had planned to come to Monte Carlo with me and Erin was going to stay with her friend for a few nights until we returned on the Sunday. Then the following Tuesday I was booked in for the op.

There were a lot of scans to fit in on the Monday and Tuesday, but I managed to do it and, on Wednesday Steve and I flew to Monte Carlo where, despite everything, we actually had a fabulous time. I felt OK after seeing Mr Kissin. It clearly wasn't good news that the cancer was back, but he seemed confident that surgery and radiotherapy would deal with it, which was reassuring.

Steve and I enjoyed our fantastic hotel and sunbathed by the pool every day, and the show was great too. I managed not to think about the cancer until I was lying in bed at night when my mind would wander and I'd start doing my 'What if?' thing. What if it wasn't that straightforward? What if it had spread?

Steve was great at saying all the right things. 'It's one lump. They're going to take it out, then you're going to have radiotherapy and that's going to be it. All your scans are going to be clear,' he kept telling me. Whether he actually believed that or if he was just saying it to keep my spirits up, I don't know. But, unusually for me, I didn't believe it. Not this time. Deep, deep down inside I knew it was more than that and I felt overwhelmed by this terrible feeling of desperation. No one else would have known, but when I was alone in the bath or the shower I'd think, 'Please God, let things be OK.'

We flew back on the Sunday and that night Mr Kissin

called me at home. He'd said he'd call as soon as he had the results of my scans.

I was standing in the kitchen when I took the call, Steve and Linda were in the sitting room and Erin had gone to bed.

'I need you to come in and see me tomorrow,' he said.

'But I'm having my operation on Tuesday,' I replied, confused.

'You're not having the operation now because the cancer has spread,' he said.

For a split second I thought I was going to be sick. I felt this horrible cocktail of emotions – horror, fear, anger.

I tried to compose myself. 'Can you tell me where it's spread?' I asked.

'No, we can't discuss it over the phone, Bernie. If you come in tomorrow you'll see me and Dr Houston together,' he said.

'OK, I'll see you then,' I said, replacing the receiver.

Steve came into the kitchen just as I'd put the phone down and he could tell immediately from the expression on my face that something was badly wrong.

'The cancer has spread, Steve,' I said. I can't even explain how devastated he looked. It broke my heart. I felt so guilty for dragging him and Erin through all of this with me. 'Maybe I should just disappear to some desert island so you and Erin don't have to deal with this,' I muttered. We stood in the kitchen, holding each other for a few minutes, then went to find Linda to deliver the news. I'd already confided in her about the lump, but she was totally shocked when I explained that the cancer had spread.

'Where has it spread to?' she asked.

'He wouldn't tell me over the phone,' I replied. 'I just hope it's not in my brain, that would be sort of awful.'

'No, God no! It won't be your brain, Bernie.'

Linda and I had both battled breast cancer, but I don't think either of us could get our heads around the idea of the disease invading our bodies – that was what happened to other people.

The following day Steve and I went to the Royal Surrey for my appointment. Mark Kissin and Stephen Houston were both there, and so was my lovely breast care nurse, Helen.

'How much do you know, Bernie?' asked Dr Houston.

'Well, I know that the cancer is back and that it's spread. That's all,' I replied nervously.

'Right well, there's a little bit in your lungs and your liver and your bones . . . and your brain.'

Bang! Bang! Bang! Every word felt like a bullet. I wanted to scream at him, 'Stop! Tell me where it isn't!' But I just sat there, completely stunned. I'd made such a brilliant recovery, better than most women I'd been told. So what happened?

Steve broke the silence: 'You said you'd got it all,' he said quietly.

Dr Houston explained the thing about cancer is that it can hide and come back at any time. It was almost like it had sneezed and a tiny bit of it had scattered everywhere.

I felt like I was floating above the situation, looking down on all of us gathered in that office. I had never experienced a feeling like it before.

'It's incurable, Bernie,' Dr Houston went on. 'But it's treatable.'

Another bullet. Then I heard myself asking the dreaded question you hear in movies. 'Well, how long have I got?'

'We're talking years,' he said. 'But not long years.'

What did that mean? That could mean literally anything. But at the time I didn't push him. There was a part of me that didn't want to know.

'I'm so sorry, Bernie,' continued Dr Houston. 'But it is treatable with drugs, that's the good thing, so I'm going off now to work out a plan for you.'

Once he'd left, Mr Kissin sat forward in his chair and took my hands in his.

'He's got to give you the worst-case scenario,' he said gently. 'I have people who have been on those drugs for fifteen years. Now that's a long time. This will be fine, you know.' He got up and put his arms around me, and that's when I broke down.

'I don't want to die,' I said, sobbing in his arms.

'We're not going to let you die; not for a long time. There are things we can do.'

He was just amazing. He didn't have to be involved with my treatment at all after that because he was a surgeon and now my treatment would be drugs only, which is Stephen Houston's job as an oncologist. But he told me: 'I'm going to stay involved all the way through and be your guardian angel. I'm going to be watching over you.'

What a thing to say.

Then he left and it was just Steve, Helen and me in the room.

'I think I'm going to be sick,' said Steve. The blood had drained from his face and he was deathly pale.

'Open the window and just breathe in some fresh air,' said Helen.

'There's a special garden area that's good to visit when you've had this kind of news,' she added, pointing out the window.

I knew the garden. It's beautiful. I used to see people sitting in it and think, 'Poor them!' and wonder what terrible news had driven them there. I never thought I'd end up in that garden myself.

'Do you want to go? There will be nobody there; it'll be quiet.'

Where else could we go? I didn't want to be with other people, so Steve and I walked together in silence to the garden.

I cried a lot in that garden, and I was ranting and raving too, shouting, 'This shouldn't be happening! Why is this happening to me?' I was filled with rage and needed to let it out. Steve was upset, too, but he kept trying to find something positive to say.

'You're that girl, Bernie,' he said, looking straight into my eyes. 'You can be the exception to the rule, that miracle case. Why shouldn't you be? If anyone is capable of it, you are.'

I had to go back into the hospital to talk to Helen about my drugs, so Steve and I made our way back inside.

'Do you want to come back tomorrow and pick up your medication?' she asked. 'It's going to take a while to get it all together.'

'I don't care! I want it now.' I didn't want to waste another minute. I wanted those cancer-killing drugs in my body as soon as possible.

I had to leave Steve with Helen while one of the other nurses did some basic tests and, when I came back, she pulled me to one side.

'Steve really lost it when you went, Bernie,' she told me. Apparently he was inconsolable. I guess he hadn't wanted to have a meltdown in front of me. But he needed to let it out, too.

After we got home that day I kept bursting into tears because I just couldn't get my head around what was happening to me. Every time I thought about what Dr Houston had said, it just seemed unbelievable and unfair.

'I'm supposed to live to ninety-nine like Auntie Lily,' I screamed at Steve. I'd almost said to Dr Houston, 'Look, there must have been a mistake. I'm Auntie Lily!'

But I wasn't; I was Bernie. This was now part of my story and I hated it.

I was incredibly low for about a week. I was filled with so much anger and when Erin was at school I'd cry and rant and scream and shout. I needed to do it.

Steve was wonderful. He'd taken my initial diagnosis much worse than I had, but this time I was the one in a really bad place. Don't get me wrong, he did his share of ranting and crying too. But he rallied quicker and he was comforting and positive.

'Look, this has happened. What are you going to do about it? That's what it's about now,' he said.

So I began by telling my family that the cancer had

returned. Linda already knew because she'd been staying with us. And I called her on the way back from the appointment with Mark Kissin and Stephen Houston to tell her where it had spread. I knew she'd be anxiously waiting at home.

When I told her the cancer was in my brain I heard a sharp intake of breath on the other end of the line. She knew the thought of that had terrified me.

'Oh my God, your brain, Bernie?'

'Yes, but it's treatable,' I said, trying to hold it together.

To be honest, it was exhausting telling people and saying those words over and over again – 'It's treatable . . . there are lots of new drugs . . . loads of people live with it' – all the stuff Mark and Stephen had said to me at the hospital.

I phoned Maureen and Coleen, and Maureen agreed to tell Anne, Denise and Tommy. I spoke to my brother Brian though, who was devastated, and I really wished I could have been with him instead of on the other end of the phone. I wanted him to see me so he could see I was OK. I wanted to put my arms around him and tell him everything was going to be fine. Even though he's older than I am, he's kind of like my baby brother sometimes. He's such a lovely guy and he loves all of us girls so much. 'We're going to blast it with drugs, Brian,' I said defiantly.

Telling Erin was another thing altogether. It was different this time – the diagnosis was much harder to put a positive spin on. How could I tell her it had spread throughout my body and was in my brain? How could I tell her it was incurable? There is nothing positive to say about that.

Once again, her birthday was coming up – she was going to be thirteen – and I didn't want to spoil it for her. Steve and I talked it over and we decided to tell her the cancer had come back in my breast and that I'd be taking pills to treat it. But that's all we were going to tell her for the time being. I still needed time to get used to the news myself and let it sink in. I wasn't sure at that stage if I wanted to go public with it; I just wanted to live with it for a while before making any other decisions.

I gave Erin the example of our friend who's HIV positive and another friend who's diabetic, and explained how they were kept alive on drugs and that's what would be happening for me. We played it down and she accepted it really well. 'OK Mum, thanks for telling me,' was all she said. My heart broke for Erin, but I didn't show her that I was upset. The last thing I wanted to do was send her into a panic.

After a week of feeling very bad and doing a lot of 'Why me?' ranting and raving, I'm glad to say the real Bernie kicked in again. I thought back to what Steve had said in the hospital garden, about being that 'miracle girl' and being the exception to the rule. One day I just thought, 'I can't feel like this forever – I could have another ten or fifteen years of life.' My friend with HIV had been living with it for twenty-five years. Why couldn't I be like him? I needed to find that positivity I'd had when I was first diagnosed. I needed to fight back. So I latched on to the one word that Dr Houston had said that was positive: 'treatable'. He could have said 'terminal' and told me I had six months to live. That would have been a lot worse. I started telling myself that every cancer patient is different. It's a bit like having a baby – each woman's experience is unique and no two births are the same. To fight this cancer, it was important that I focused just on my own story.

Since being diagnosed with breast cancer in 2010, my philosophy had been, 'I'm living with it, not dying from it,' and that was even more relevant now. And, if you dig deep, it is possible to think like that. Without wishing to be too dramatic, we're all going to die one day, it's just that I've had an early warning. I always knew I was going to die, I just didn't know when. And I still don't.

Being told you have incurable cancer is a very hard concept to get your head around and each person has to find their own way of living with that knowledge. Getting on with living and being positive is just the way I decided to approach it in the weeks and months following the diagnosis. It's not in my nature to sit around dwelling on death. I'm naturally optimistic and somehow that positivity always rises to the surface – it's the only way I know how to be. It's the only way I could deal with such a bleak prognosis.

Some people might say I was in denial, but I knew all the details and all the facts and figures. I took the bloody tablets every day! But I did my best not to think about it. At bedtime it would wander into my mind or when I was taking my tablets, or if somebody asked me how I was doing. All of a sudden, I'd think, 'Shit! I've got incurable cancer!' But the rest of the time, I got on with my life and took things day by day. That's how I was able to live with it.

*　*　*

At home, things settled down, which was good because I wanted to keep things as normal as possible – for myself, but mostly for Erin. As any mum knows, whatever happens in your life – good or bad – your first thought is always: how will this affect my child? I wanted to shield Erin as much as possible from the worst aspects of my illness. I couldn't make it go away, I couldn't tell her truthfully that things were going to be OK, but I could try to keep her life the same. I was determined to do that. And it was important that she looked at me and saw I was coping and that I was OK.

Her birthday that year was hideous for Steve and me though – sorry Erin! She wanted a big party with a DJ because she was becoming a teenager. I had to face up to the fact my little girl was growing up – there would be no cake, no pass the parcel, just sixty teens and pre-teens going nuts! She invited all her Facebook friends and they were little buggers. Steve and I spent the whole night trying to keep them in line.

'Never again, Erin!' I told her the next day. 'OK, Mum,' she said. I think even she realised it had been a bit crazy.

We got a video made of the night for her, which I reckon she's watched once and it cost about £150! But, the important thing is, she loved the party at the time and life is all about those moments.

At work, too, I was determined for things not to change. It was easier to carry on working this time around because I wasn't on intravenous chemotherapy – I was taking an oral chemo drug along with Herceptin. The medication made me feel tired at first and I was warned my hair could thin but that it wouldn't fall out this time, which I was relieved about.

I carried on with *Chicago* and didn't tell anyone on the cast that the cancer had returned, apart from one friend, Nettie, who was the lead trumpet player. I knew I could trust her to keep it a secret. She'd been through breast cancer herself and had undergone a mastectomy and reconstruction, but the reconstruction had gone wrong so she sued the hospital and won. On the day she found out she'd be getting compensation, she texted me to offer me all the money to go to America and pay for the latest cancer drugs.

I texted her back right away: 'Oh my God, Nettie, you stupid bitch, don't be so silly, there's no way I'm taking your money! But thank you!'

It was so incredibly touching. Since getting cancer I've realised how many lovely people are out there. Of course there are some shits, but they're mostly nice!

Nettie was very inspiring. She's an amazing trumpet player, but she lost all her confidence after her cancer treatment and almost gave up playing. When she joined *Chicago* she hadn't played for ages and wasn't sure she wanted to do it so, at her first rehearsal, she decided to play the first ten bars of *Annie* instead of *Chicago* to see how people reacted. 'I thought, if they get funny with me, fuck 'em, I'm going home,' she told me afterwards.

But the music director and everyone else at the rehearsal thought she was hilarious and fell about laughing, so she decided to give it a go. She's absolutely mental, just like me, which is why we got on so well.

I also had to tell the producer David Ian because every

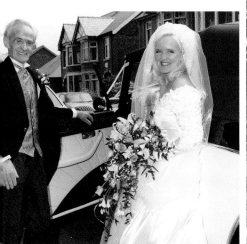

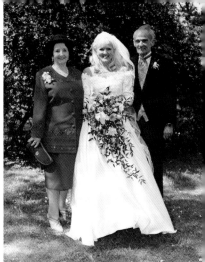

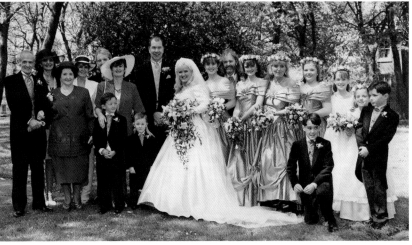

Steve and I were married on
25 May 1996. I wanted a big
white wedding and the day
was everything I hoped for.
Steve is the love of my life and
has been my rock.

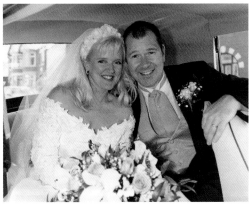

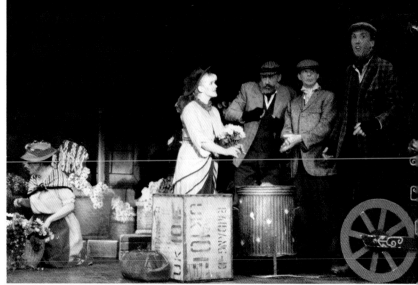

I've done so many shows over the years but this was one of my favourites, I played Eliza Doolittle in *My Fair Lady*.

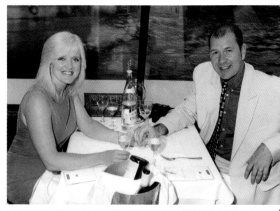

Steve and I celebrated our first anniversary in Paris 1997.

The whole family came together in Blackpool for my fortieth birthday, which was a brilliant party!

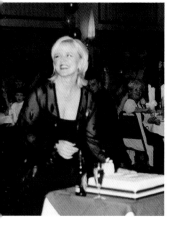

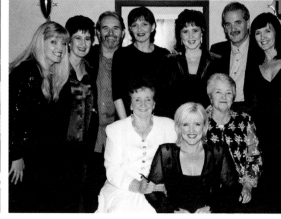

Family has always been very important to me. Here are my mum and dad, with my mum's sister Auntie Teresa, who was like a second mum to me, and her husband Jim.

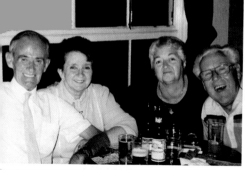

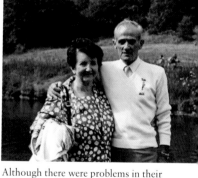

Although there were problems in their relationship, my parents did love each other deeply. Here they are visiting Denise in Scarborough.

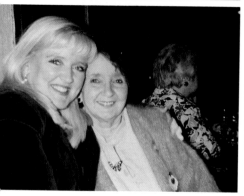

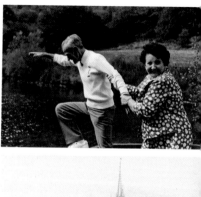

My mum was a wonderful person – she was kind, beautiful and had a brilliant sense of humour. We were always very close.

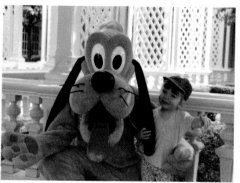

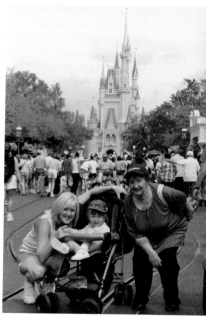

Erin adores Disney, and we have had so many happy holidays in Florida. Here is Erin with me, Mum, and Pluto!

My Brookside family – the Murrays. From left to right we are Ray Quinn, Neil Caple, Steven Fletcher, me and Katy Lamont. I loved being Diane!

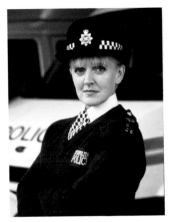

I spent a brilliant three years playing Sergeant Sheelagh Murphy on *The Bill*.

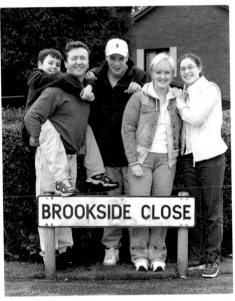

Having a ball at the National Television Awards in 2004, where we won the Most Popular Drama award for *The Bill*.

Popstar to Operastar was a brilliant experience – I got all the way to the final but was beaten by just half a point by Darius Campbell from *Pop Idol*.

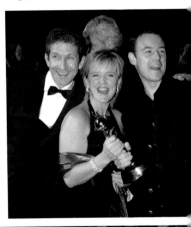

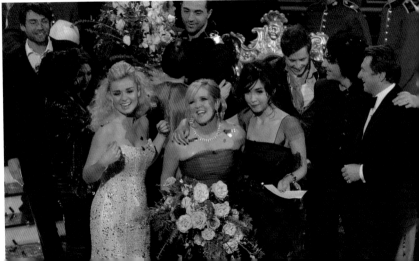

Erin loves her aunties and we often go on holiday together. Here we are with Maureen and Linda in Spain.

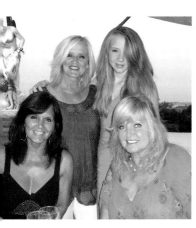

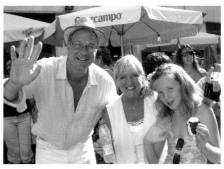

Steve, Erin and I in Malaga in 2009.

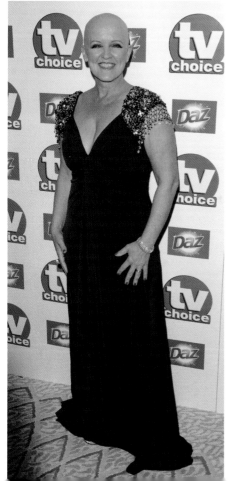

I decided not to wear my wig for the TV Choice Awards in 2010. I wanted to show solidarity with all the women fighting breast cancer. I'm very glad I did it because afterwards I received so many messages of thanks and people telling me that I had helped someone in their family.

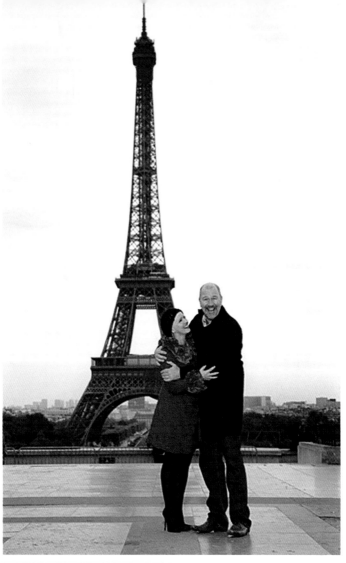

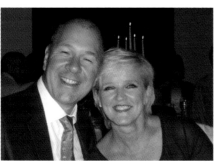

In October 2010 Steve and I visited Paris, where we had celebrated our first wedding anniversary. He has been there for me through everything, and I couldn't ask for a more loving or supportive husband.

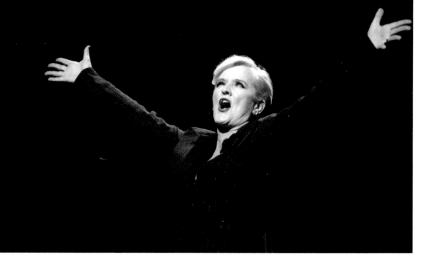

was appearing in *Chicago* when I found out that my cancer had come back and that it was incurable. But I still carried on with the show, had a blast and the cast and crew were all brilliant.

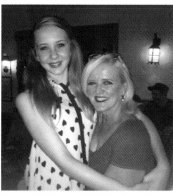

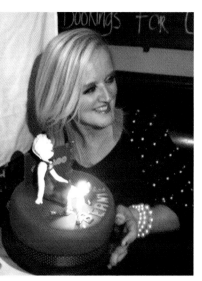

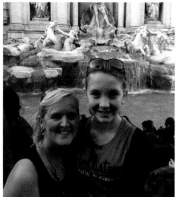

I was on tour with *Chicago* in Belfast on my 52nd birthday. Steve and Erin came out to surprise me, and I had a special Mama Morton birthday cake – it was fantastic!

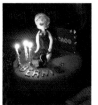

Another wonderful family moment was our holiday to Rome in February 2012, just a few months before I found out the cancer had returned. Steve, Erin and I were joined by Linda, my brother Brian and his wife Annie.

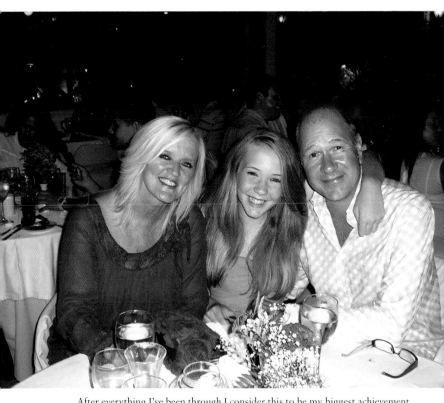

After everything I've been through I consider this to be my biggest achievement, my wonderful family.

three weeks I needed to go to the Royal Surrey for blood tests and to get a drip to strengthen my bones. Treatment was usually a Friday and I had two shows on a Friday, which I would have to miss.

Although we'd known each other for years and had dated in the past, this was business and he didn't owe me anything. I'm sure he could have sued me or terminated my contract if he'd wanted to, but of course he was amazing.

'Whatever you need, Bernie,' he said, when I broke the news. 'If you need a driver, take my car whenever you need it. And don't worry, we won't be deducting any money from your fee for time off.'

I've been very fortunate in my career to be surrounded by some of the best people in the business, and David Ian is right at the top of that list. He understood that what was happening to me was real. Showbiz didn't matter.

He made it possible for me to continue working, which I desperately needed to do because I felt like Bernie at work. Once I was all done up in my Mama Morton costume and stage make-up, I felt like me again.

Mentally and emotionally I needed work more than ever. I would have felt lost without it. When I was first diagnosed it was right to stop working so I could put all my energy into fighting the disease and recovering from surgery. But now my cancer was incurable, what was I going to do if I didn't work – sit around the house feeling like Cancer Girl for the rest of my days? I needed to feel like my life was carrying on. I needed the distraction. And I'll always be grateful to David for making it easy for me.

So I carried on touring with the show that summer and

Steve and Erin joined me during the school holidays. We went to Dublin, Truro and Torquay, where Erin learned to bodyboard. We had a nice time and the audiences were great, so it all helped to lift me and keep me positive.

I also had a week's holiday to take, so we decided to go to our apartment in Mijas, which is a gorgeous little old Spanish town on the Costa del Sol. Maureen and Linda came with us and rented somewhere nearby, and we had a fantastic time. We walked on the beach and had long lunches over chilled glasses of wine, and laughed so much, which they say is the best medicine. It was bliss.

Physically, I felt really well. I had scans coming up towards the end of July, so until then there was nothing to do except carry on taking the pills and attend my regular check-ups.

In July, Steve and I found ourselves in a scary and, sadly, all too familiar situation – sitting outside my oncologist Stephen Houston's office, waiting for the results of my scans. For the past week I'd had all these questions running through my mind: 'Has the cancer spread? Is it bigger? Is it still treatable?'

The hospital was so busy that day and we were kept waiting for nearly three hours, which only added to our agony. Just as I was about to start pulling my hair out, Olga, one of the breast care nurses, came over and sat beside us. 'You'll be going in soon, Bernie,' she said, clearly aware of how anxious I was. 'But it's all good,' she added, patting my hand reassuringly before leaving us. My ears pricked up immediately. 'Did you hear that, Steve? She said it was all good,' I said excitedly. 'She wouldn't have said that unless there was some good news.'

'I know, but let's just wait to see what Dr Houston has to say,' replied Steve, cautiously. He obviously didn't want me getting my hopes up, only for them to be dashed two minutes later.

To be honest, over the previous few weeks, I'd been clinging on to the possibility that things had stayed the same, that the cancer hadn't got bigger or spread anywhere else. That was my biggest hope.

'Well,' said Dr Houston when we were finally seated in his office. 'The cancer has gone from your brain.'

'What?' said Steve, turning to look at me in disbelief.

'But it's incurable, isn't it?' I added, unable to take in what Dr Houston had just told us.

'Look, I can't explain it, but it's gone from your brain and it's also shrunk, quite a lot, everywhere else. There are still some lesions in your lungs, but some have gone completely. So, in other words, the treatment is working.'

We were elated and wanted to go home immediately and crack open a bottle of champagne. It was the most exciting news and much, much more than we'd hoped for. However, I had to spend the rest of that day in hospital, waiting for my next lot of tablets, so by the time Steve and I got home we were too exhausted to bother with the champers, even though we had a nice bottle of Bolly chilling in the fridge!

It was the first bit of good news we'd heard in a long time and I was determined to hang on to it. Over the next few days I started to ponder the idea of going public with it. It was still only my closest family and friends who knew that my cancer had returned. I hadn't even told Erin that it had spread.

I thought about other people struggling with cancer who didn't have a Steve for support or anyone close to fall back on, for that matter. If I could share my good news, it might give them hope. I also thought it might give Erin a boost to see me being so positive publicly. I'm so glad we waited to tell her that the cancer had spread because now we could do it with a positive slant – I could tell her honestly that the tablets were working and that the cancer had gone from my brain.

So, a few days after we'd seen Dr Houston, Steve and I sat down with her and broke the news. In typical Erin style, she handled it calmly and with incredible maturity.

'Why didn't you tell me it had spread before, Mum?' she asked.

'Erin, I just didn't think it was something a thirteen-year-old needed to live with. It's hard enough for me to live with it!'

'Mum, you know you can tell me everything. I want to know everything,' she said. So that was me told!

Although I'd been positive over the summer, the news the medication was working gave me a major boost. I started necking those pills with joy! They did bring some side effects, but it was manageable stuff. I got mouth ulcers again, but thankfully it was eight this time, not twenty-five! And the skin on my feet started to peel, so the soles of my feet were sore, which did become a bit of a problem on stage. But I told the lovely wardrobe mistress at *Chicago* – who still didn't know about my cancer – that my shoes were uncomfortable and she found these amazing gel pads that hook on to one of your toes and cushion the ball of your foot when you're wearing heels. They were a life-saver! It's amazing how little things like that can make a huge difference to how you feel and cope with things day to day.

The drugs were powerful, but still preferable to intravenous chemo. And apparently I was given tablets because intravenous chemo doesn't reach your brain. However, at my last appointment Dr Houston had lowered my dose of chemo slightly because of the mouth ulcers and peeling skin on my feet.

'But I don't want you to do that. The tablets are working!' I'd told him, slightly panicked. I was worried that a lower dose wouldn't be as effective. I figured a few mouth ulcers were a small price to pay for still being alive.

'Look, the thing about this treatment is that it's all about the quality of life,' he explained. 'If you can't eat, or drink or sleep because you have mouth ulcers, that's no quality of life. I'm only going to lower it by a couple of milligrams. Trust me.'

In October *Chicago* hit Belfast. My fifty-second birthday was on Wednesday 17. Steve and Erin couldn't come with me because she was in school and I don't like taking her away from her studies. I was sad they wouldn't be with me, but I decided to have a big birthday meal at a local restaurant with the cast. Jamie Baughan, who played Mr Cellophane, and our fabulous company manager Leighton organised it all and sorted out the menu. I was staying with a friend of Linda's – William Caulfield and his lovely partner Mark – so she came over for the week too, which was lovely for me. The night before my birthday, I arranged to meet Linda and William in a bar after the show. When I arrived I spotted Linda straight away, standing at the bar.

'I've got you a glass of wine,' she said. 'William's over there; let's go and sit down.' And as I walked over to where William was supposed to be, Steve and Erin were sitting at the table. I started crying immediately!

'My God! You liars!' I screamed, hugging them both. I was so happy to see them.

It turned out that Steve had booked the three of us into a lovely hotel for two nights and had even been in touch with Jamie to say they'd be coming along to my birthday dinner. Linda had packed an overnight bag for me with clothes, toiletries and all my medication and delivered it to the hotel. And Steve had arranged lunch in the hotel restaurant for the family the next day.

I'd just sat down to take a sip of wine and get over the shock when I saw a figure coming towards us – it was Maureen! 'Jesus! What's going on, you lot?' I squealed. 'I won't die of bloody cancer; I'll die of a heart attack!'

I'm the one who normally does surprises in our family and organises all the parties, so I was completely blown away by what they'd done.

The next day, after the show, we all had a fantastic meal with the cast, and William and Mark who I'd been staying with brought along a special *Chicago* birthday cake they'd had made in Belfast with Mama Morton sitting on top. It was one of my best birthdays ever and

I was deeply touched by the effort everyone had made. Times like that are what life is all about and they're a reminder that it's people that matter, not money or fame or showbiz or bullshit!

After that, *Chicago* rolled on to Woking, Preston and then Derry. My wonderful producer David allowed me to stay at home the week the show was in Derry because I'd done an interview with the *Sunday Mirror* revealing that my cancer was back and it was coming out on 28 October. I wanted to be with Erin when the story broke just in case she was upset by anything.

My *Chicago* colleagues still didn't know about my cancer, so I decided to send each member of the cast and crew a personal email on the Saturday night so they didn't have to find out by reading it in the paper. If I'd been in Derry, I would have called them all together and told them face to face. Only my immediate family were in the picture, so I also had to send emails to other relatives and friends who didn't know. There were a lot of shocked people that Saturday night.

It was quite cathartic doing that piece for the paper and it was a good way to show all the people I cared about that I was being strong and positive. In the piece I said my next goal was Erin's twenty-first birthday and that I intended to be there 'with bells on', which I'm sure was nice for her to read.

On the Monday it was back to work in Crawley and I had to face the *Chicago* cast and crew. So at the sound-check I made a little announcement. 'Just act normal everyone. I've known for months about the cancer, so it's not news to me,' I said, hearing gasps around the room.

'But I didn't want anybody to know because I hadn't told Erin the full story and I didn't know how I was going to cope myself. And I'm sorry I didn't get a chance to tell you in person.

'But I'm going to be here for a long, long time to come, so I don't want any pity and if I see any of you looking at me with big sad eyes, you can all fuck off!'

They all laughed and clapped and were totally amazing, as I knew they would be. Once they all knew, I carried on using humour to cope at work and to diffuse tensions. Sometimes if there was a row going on or someone was having a go at me, I'd pipe up, 'Um, you can't be horrible to me, I've got cancer, you know.'

'Oh, bloody hell, not the cancer card again!' they'd all sigh.

It wasn't long before the cast and crew started calling Nettie and me the Chemo Sisters, and if we happened to leave work together, some smartarse would bellow, 'Cancer has left the building!'

It was funny and it was exactly how I wanted them to behave around me. I was determined to live with this cancer, so we had to get to a place where people knew how to treat me – and that attitude had to come from me. I know there are people who probably wouldn't appreciate that sort of humour but that's just the way I am.

13
HELLO COUGH, GOODBYE *CHICAGO*
....

In November I hit a bit of a wall. I developed a cough, which I just couldn't shift. There were a lot of winter viruses doing the rounds and I assumed I couldn't shake it off because my immune system was low. I carried on with the tour, though, travelling to Canterbury and Glasgow, but most of the time I couldn't go on stage because I was coughing too much to sing or say my lines.

I found it all really devastating, but I tried to keep my spirits up by continuing to show up for work and hoping that I'd be able to go on. Most people would have stayed at home and tried to get better, but I've never been the sort of person to take sick days. I've got an insanely strong work ethic, which I think I inherited from my parents, and I wanted to show willing because David Ian had been so good to me. I didn't want to let him down. So I flew up to Glasgow and stayed in digs, and I drove to Canterbury from Weybridge every day just in case I could sing, and every day I was sent home after the soundcheck.

The tour was ending its run at the Theatre Royal in

Plymouth on 1 December. I travelled down there on 26 November, hoping I'd make it on stage at some point that week, but my cough wasn't getting any better. I'd really wanted to go out with a bang, but it looked like it would be more of a whimper!

My cough had started to play on my mind. I had cancer in my lungs after all; only a small amount, but I did start to worry that the cough was connected to the disease. My voice meant everything to me and not being able to perform was killing my spirit. So while I was in Plymouth I paid privately to see an ear, nose and throat specialist and had a camera put down my throat.

The doctor couldn't find any nodules and my airways were clear, but one of my vocal cords wasn't working properly, which was a real worry.

'It might have become weakened because you've been coughing so much,' said the doctor. 'Or it could be something more serious.'

He explained that something further down could be pressing on it – maybe fibrous tissue from my operation or a tumour. I would have to wait for further tests.

I'd been so positive, but not being able to speak or sing was really getting me down. And the constant coughing was exhausting. One night Nettie and I got back to our digs after a night out and I just let rip. 'God, Nettie, this is getting to me,' I said when we were sitting on the sofa having a drink. 'Not only do I have cancer, which I'm dealing with, but now my voice is gone, I can't speak for coughing and I can't do my job. Jesus Christ! Give me a break!'

There haven't been many days when I've felt sorry for

myself, but that was one of them. I could fire off at Nettie – she'd struggled with similar feelings herself and she understood my frustration and how it feels not to be in control of your own body.

You have to let it out sometimes. Although I always tried hard to find something positive in whatever my illness threw at me, I never put my head in the sand and pretended it wasn't happening. I was always 100% on top of my scans and treatment. And of course there were times when I did scream the place down, and rant and rave – usually to Steve or my sisters. I talked about it when I needed to talk about it, but I was also aware that it's hard knowing what to say back to me and I didn't want the conversation to always be about cancer. That wouldn't be helpful for me and it would be boring for everyone else.

I didn't like people assuming I wanted advice or information. One day I got sent a load of pamphlets and books about how to live with cancer from one of the charities, which I hadn't asked for, and that annoyed me. Anyone who's been where I've been will understand that – if I'd wanted help I would have asked for it. I started to read one of the books and it really upset me, so I ended up flinging the lot in the bin. I knew someone was just trying to be nice, but it wasn't what I wanted.

On another occasion, when I was in Glasgow with *Chicago*, someone left a figurine of Saint Peregrine, the patron saint of cancer, along with a prayer book and a prayer card in my dressingroom, and I'm not religious at all. Again, it was a lovely thought, but it felt a bit strange that someone had just left it there.

I wasn't the sort of person to revel in my illness. There

are people who love to talk in great detail about their condition – maybe that's their way of dealing with it, but it's not mine. One time when I was at the Royal Surrey for my bone cannula drip, I got chatting to a woman in her thirties who was being treated for breast cancer. She was a mum with two young kids under three.

'What are you here for – have you had breast cancer?' she enquired.

'Yes, I did have breast cancer,' I replied. 'I had chemo and a mastectomy, which all went brilliantly and I was fine.'

'So what are you in for now?' she pushed.

'You really don't want to know that. Just know that I recovered really well from the breast cancer and hopefully you will too.'

I didn't want to go into the fact the cancer had come back and it had spread – why would that have been helpful for her? I always wanted to focus on the good stuff.

There were times when people's staggering insensitivity gave me a laugh, though.

'Yeah, my mum had what you've got and she died,' someone once said.

'Um, thanks!'

I also had one lady say, 'You know, my daughter was your age and she died of cancer.'

'Jesus!'

I really didn't want to know other people's bad stories. I had enough bad news of my own to deal with! And, I know this sounds corny, but I wanted to have my own journey. I wanted to know the medical facts about my own condition and what I could do to help myself, but that was it. I felt it was vital for me to maintain my positive attitude and my energy. One of the first things Mr Kissin advised me never to do was Google anything related to my illness and I can honestly say that I didn't. Most people who Google health problems and have nothing wrong with them come away thinking they're going to die of some horrible disease, so can you imagine what you'd come up with if you actually had cancer?

I won't lie; of course I had my private moments of despair, lying in my bed alone in the dark, thinking about what might happen, about dying from cancer. But every time I felt myself slipping into those depths, I told myself that kind of thinking wasn't going to help me. Sometimes it would catch me first thing in the morning. I'd wake up feeling really happy like I've always done and then the horrible realisation would hit me and I'd think, 'Oh yeah, there's that. I have cancer.' Those moments were the hardest.

But generally I think I coped really well and work helped me immeasurably. I knew lying on the sofa at home would make me feel sicker and I didn't want to behave like an ill person.

During the last week of *Chicago*, Steve was totally brilliant because he just let me be myself. My cough was so bad that I could barely hold a conversation with him on the phone and I'm sure he just wanted me to get in the car and drive home to be with him and Erin, but he didn't put any pressure on me. He knows me inside out and he understood it was important for me to have that sense of 'business as usual'.

I called Steve three times a day. The morning after my outburst to Nettie, I was feeling pretty low and said to him, 'Look, my throat is really bad, so I might come home tomorrow. I'm just lying around here and I probably won't get to do any more shows.'

I guess most guys would have said, 'Yeah, I think you should come back now,' especially as I was about to go into rehearsals for panto in Eastbourne just a couple of days after *Chicago* finished.

'Well, why not give it another day?' Steve suggested. 'See how you feel when you wake up tomorrow. Your throat might improve; but even if it doesn't, you might feel better sticking it out and being with everyone at the end. You might regret it otherwise.'

And that's what I love about him. It was so generous of him to make me feel OK about being away from home. And Erin, God love her, was the same. 'No, you should stay in Plymouth, Mum,' she insisted. 'Finish off the tour, even if you can't go on stage.'

She's so grown-up and responsible, which makes me very proud.

Both of them were used to me touring – I'd been doing it for ten years since having Erin – and I always recognised that it was much harder on Steve than it was on me. I had the best of both worlds, really. When I was away I didn't have to get up early for the school run, I could go out drinking with my friends after the show and lie in bed if I wanted to, I got to see new places all the time and I was doing what I loved most: singing. It's much, much harder for the person at home, as most women will appreciate, keeping it all together and following the same routine day after day. I don't think I would have been as generous as Steve – he's been absolutely outstandingly unbelievable! I'm sure if he'd been the one on tour I would have been moaning all the time and wanting to know where he'd been and who he was with and when he was going to call next. But Steve's attitude was always, 'Go out for a drink and enjoy yourself. Don't worry about phoning, I'll speak to you tomorrow.' He never gave me a hard time.

Don't get me wrong, he's not perfect and he can also drive me insane! He's very opinionated and set in his ways and he can be terribly grumpy, especially in the morning. And because my glass is always half full and his is generally half empty, I'm constantly trying to pick him up. So we've had our problems, like all couples, but we get each other and we respect each other. And if we have been going through a tough time, instead of just giving up and saying, 'Screw this, I'm off,' we've both persevered because the good times far outweigh the bad ones.

In the end, I didn't perform at all during that final week of *Chicago*, but Steve and Erin were right – I was still happy to be there with the cast and crew at the end. It sounds a bit soft really, but over the past ten months I'd felt really loved and cared for by the people on that show. And there was great camaraderie between us all, too. When you're away from home, you have to make the best of it, so it was a godsend to be working with such a great bunch of people. I definitely made friends for life on that tour.

On one of the last nights we had a fancy-dress party and I went as a nun, which I thought was funny because

The Nolans always had that reputation of being sweet and innocent. And of course all the people on *Chicago* thought it was inspired because they know I love to have a drink and party – not very nun-like! Everyone made a huge effort with their costumes. Two of the dancers went as bananas, Stefan Booth went as Mr T and Nettie had made a ballet dancer's tutu out of white bin-bags!

We hired a room in a lovely bar and when that closed at midnight, we walked to another place nearby called Bang Bang and most people got horribly drunk. I managed to keep things at the tipsy level, but the dancers were wrecked and there were people lying all over the floor. Most of us had no clue how to get home. It was carnage! Nettie and I shared a taxi back to our digs. She was smart, though, and had brought some jeans to change into for the journey home. I, on the other hand, was still in my nun's habit. I'll never forget the look on the cab driver's face as I bundled myself into the back of his car, swearing like a trouper because I'd tripped over my costume.

'Shit! I nearly broke my bloody neck!'

I guess he doesn't see many drunken nuns! It was a very funny night.

The following evening, our last night, the company manager Leighton arranged a farewell meal at an Italian restaurant and there were thirty-seven of us there. I gave everyone little presents, which I'd been ordering on-line for the previous five or six weeks and getting engraved with personal messages. I think they were all gobsmacked and really touched. But their friendship and support had meant such a lot to me during a really tough time in my life.

I made a little speech, thanking everyone for their kindness and support, and Nettie got up and said a few words too. She talked a bit about breast cancer and how important it was to be vigilant for any unusual changes – typical Nettie!

After the meal, about eight of us headed to a casino and I didn't leave until 4 a.m. We had a brilliant laugh. I ended up leaving Nettie there – she rolled in about 6.30 a.m.! Steve had told me to go out, forget about all the bad stuff and have a great time, so that's exactly what I did. But I was really going to miss everyone and I was really going to miss the show.

14
THE SHOW CAN'T GO ON

....

'What the fuck am I doing here?' I said, burying my face in my hands. 'I should be at home with my family.'

I was sitting alone in my digs in Eastbourne, wishing to God I hadn't signed up for panto. I was in the first week of rehearsals for *Sleeping Beauty* at the Devonshire Park Theatre and I was playing Carabosse, the wicked fairy. I'd brought a few personal things to make my accommodation feel more homely and comfy – photographs of Steve and Erin, a cushion and a blanket for the sofa – but none of it was having the desired effect. I suddenly missed home a lot and Weybridge felt a million miles away.

I kept being gripped by this horrible feeling of panic that I should be with my husband and daughter. At the same time, I was also terrified that if I didn't carry on doing the things I always did, I would feel my illness even more keenly and life would change, which wasn't what I wanted. That's what having this illness does to you – it messes with your head.

But I'd been so depressed at missing the last few weeks of *Chicago* because of my cough, I was keen to get back on stage. Unfortunately my throat wasn't getting any better; in fact it was getting worse and I was losing my voice. Fortunately, I had pre-recorded my songs for the show and had them on tape, which meant I wouldn't have to sing live during the show – I actually couldn't sing for more than a few seconds before having a coughing fit.

The cast and crew were all lovely and I'd already worked with the producer Chris Jordan, who's a great guy. They knew about my cancer and that my throat was bad, and they looked after me brilliantly. One of the dancers did my hair in a plait every night and once I had my make-up on I really looked the part – and, of course, I felt like Bernie.

As usual, I was straight in there at the first rehearsal with my cancer gags so no one would feel awkward.

'Right you lot, you can't be arsey to me because I've got cancer,' I said and they all laughed. One of the guys didn't know I was ill, though, and thought I was kidding. The next day I made another joke and he said, 'Oh, stop saying that, Bernie! That's terrible! You might get it.'

'I have got it!' I replied.

'Oh God, I'm so sorry. I didn't know,' he said, looking like he wanted the stage to open up and swallow him. 'I feel terrible now.'

'Oh, shut up! It's fine. I don't want sorry. That's not a word I want to hear. No pity, right?'

'OK, you're on.'

But although everybody was wonderful and there was a nice little pub we could escape to next door, I was feeling the strain. My heart wasn't in it. I'd had only one day off since finishing *Chicago* and panto is bloody hard work, as anyone who's ever worked on one will tell you. We had five days for rehearsals, which wasn't a lot, so it was manic and we were working until 10 p.m. every night. Chris Jordan gave me a day off to conserve some energy, which was fantastic of him, so I went home and spent the whole day just chilling out with Erin and watching rubbish telly. When I got back to Eastbourne we did the tech runs before the show opened, which involved spending all day standing around in our costumes and having really late nights.

I felt awful during our opening week and the schedule was relentless. We had three shows on a Saturday and two shows every other day. I was unbelievably tired and began to feel pretty ill. I'd lost my appetite, but I forced myself to eat because I knew I had to keep my strength up. I'd probably lost about a stone over the previous four weeks and I'd given up alcohol too, which probably contributed to the weight loss. I'd just stopped feeling like drinking and I couldn't go out and get drunk anyway because I had to stuff myself full of drugs every day. There was no way I could deal with hangovers any more.

But the most worrying symptom was that I started vomiting every night after the show. It terrified me because once your body starts rejecting the cancer medication they change it, which I didn't want to happen because Dr Houston's cocktail of drugs had been working. I was taking at least fifteen pills a day, but it was usually more than that because I was also taking painkillers regularly to cope with my back pain, which was due to the cancer in my bones. And to top it off, I'd also been necking throat pastilles after every scene because my cough was so bad. I prayed that my sickness was down to overdosing on the throat sweets and not to do with my medication.

When I went home to Weybridge on my day off, the first thing I said to Steve when I walked through the front door was, 'I don't want to do it any more.' I'd never felt defeated by work before, but physically I was wrung out.

'Pull out if you don't want to do it,' he urged, giving me a supportive hug. 'The tickets have already sold out, so I'm sure Chris will be delighted not to have to pay you!'

God, I was so tempted. I picked up the phone and called my manager Neil and explained how I'd been feeling.

'God, Bernie, we'll pull you out. Your health's more important,' he told me. 'I'll call Chris today and explain.'

'Hmm, let me think about it overnight,' I said.

When I put the phone down after talking to Neil, I was on the verge of phoning Chris myself and telling him I couldn't come back, that I'd realised it was too much for me. But I have this in-built thing in my psyche that drives me to see things through. Responsibility, loyalty, professionalism, call it whatever you want, but if I've signed a contract with someone, I don't want to let them down.

The next morning when I woke up I felt better – probably from spending the night at home – and, in typical Bernie style, thought, 'Get a grip, you silly cow. Stop being such a girl!' So I got out of bed, packed my bag, kissed Steve and Erin goodbye and drove back to Eastbourne.

Over the next few days I managed to pick myself up emotionally and physically, and I stopped throwing up. Thank God. I think I'd felt overwhelmed – I was tired and sick, and the stress of trying not to cough during the show was monumental. And I wasn't supposed to get stressed.

I only had a few days to wait before my next big hospital appointment and CT scan, and I'd be able to discuss my medication then. They'd brought the appointment forward because of my cough. They were concerned, as I was, that it was related to the cancer, and the endoscopy I'd had in Plymouth wasn't conclusive. There wasn't much I could do until I saw my own consultant and had the results of the scan.

I held on to the thought that Erin was breaking up for the school holidays in a week's time and then she and Steve would be coming to stay with me in Eastbourne. Then it wasn't long until Christmas and we'd be spending Christmas Day and Boxing Day in Weybridge before heading back to Eastbourne together. I just kept telling myself to stay strong until the end of the week.

I had also taken the following Monday – 17 December – off work to have my CT scan and I planned to take Erin Christmas shopping afterwards and pick the tree, which she was very excited about. Throughout this journey, the most important thing for me has always been to keep Erin's life as normal as possible. Any mum would feel the same. I wanted to protect Erin with every fibre of my being. I wanted to protect her childhood and her memories of me. So even though I was coughing incessantly during this time, I tried never to complain in front of her so she wouldn't feel worried or upset.

Kids are incredibly resilient and Erin is tougher than most in my opinion; even so, I worried about how she was coping. When I was tucking her in, the night before my scan, I reminded her again that it was OK to ask me questions.

'You know, if there's anything at all you want to ask me, Erin, just say . . .' I said softly.

'Mum, stop worrying and stop asking me that,' she said. 'I promise I'll tell you if there's anything I want to know.'

Then she added quietly, 'I'm doing what you're doing, Mum. I'm just pretending it's not happening and getting on with my life because what else can we do?'

Wow! I'll never know what I did to deserve such a wonderful child, but her strength spurred me on. She made everything easier for me.

Scans in themselves aren't scary, but my nerves were always jangling on the run-up to having one because you know there's no place to hide. They see right into your brain, lungs and liver – into every little part of you. If my cancer had spread or the tumours had grown bigger, it would be there in black and white for all to see. And on this occasion I knew the doctors would be checking for tumours that were pressing on my vocal cords. But I would have to wait until Friday – four long days – to get the results.

When I got back to Eastbourne the day after the scan, I sent Steve an encouraging text message: 'Whatever they tell us on Friday, it'll be OK. We will fight it together and I'll be here for a long, long time.' And I meant it.

Something had happened about a fortnight previously, which I felt a bit puzzled by. Although I'd always been one of those people who was full of *joie de vivre*, lately I'd realised I was enjoying everything much more. It was almost as if there was a little voice in my head saying, 'Enjoy every single day.' I was getting so much joy out of everything, even silly little mundane things.

I loved being at home with Steve and Erin anyway, but on my days off from the panto in Eastbourne when the three of us were sitting snuggled up on the sofa in front of the fire watching telly, I got so much pleasure from it. I began to appreciate moments like those more and more. It was as if I'd stopped to smell the roses.

I was so looking forward to Christmas. I'd helped pick out the tree, but because I had to go back to work it was up to Steve and Erin to decorate it. 'Don't forget to help your dad,' I called out to Erin as I was heading out the door to drive back to Eastbourne. 'I will, I will!' she shouted. But she didn't lift a finger. Apparently she tapped away on her laptop while Steve put up the lights and hung the baubles. Typical teenager! Steve sent me a picture of the tree and it looked gorgeous. I couldn't wait to be sitting in my living room at home with the glow of the fairy lights, a chilled glass of wine in my hand and my family around me. Linda, Maureen and Richie were coming for Christmas and my brothers Tommy and Brian were arriving on 27 December for a few days and were going to pop down to Eastbourne to see me in panto.

In the meantime, I got into the festive mood by squeezing in some Christmas shopping on my mornings off. I love buying presents much more than receiving them and I wanted this Christmas to be extra special, so I went to town on the gifts. I got Steve an Armani watch – he's fixated on watches and has tons of them. I almost bought him a Breitling watch, but it was £2,000 and I knew he'd kill me if I spent that much money! I also got him a Kenwood hand mixer and an Escoffier cookbook, which he'd wanted for ages. It was out of print so I had to search one out on-line. Erin got everything on her wish list – and tons more. She's mad about a band called The Midnight Beast, which does parodies of pop songs – she literally screams with laughter at them. She'd been to see them live and had met them backstage because Coleen's son Jake is a friend of theirs. I bought her loads of merchandise – a hat, a T-shirt and pyjamas. I got her *The Hunger Games* on DVD, two Xbox games and Keith Lemon's new movie on DVD.

I also booked us a dream holiday to Thailand in February. I'd always wanted to go there and we were all desperate for a break where we could just do nothing, eat nice food and feel the warmth of the sun on our skin. The resort I'd chosen was really luxurious – I totally blew the budget! We had a two-bedroom suite with our own pool and it looked right on to a beautiful white sandy beach. I was a bit worried it wouldn't be exciting enough for Erin and that there wouldn't be any other kids around, but she loved the idea of it.

'I just want it to be us, Mum,' she told me. 'So we can relax and swim, and not have to make friends and be nice to people.' Erin needed to de-stress too.

I'd started to think a bit about the new year and what I wanted for 2013, and I decided I didn't want to do much, other than be with my family and be a mum to Erin. I pondered the idea of doing some volunteer work for Breakthrough Breast Cancer and the stillbirth and neonatal death charity SANDS, as I'm a patron of both organisations. And I thought it might be nice to take another road trip around the country with Steve and Erin to visit family and friends. But, more than anything, I wanted to take things easy and conserve my energy for whatever battle lay ahead.

15
DON'T GIVE UP ON ME

....

OK, reality check time. As far as wake-up calls go, the one I got sitting in Stephen Houston's office on Friday 21 December was pretty massive. In a nutshell, the scan results were bad. The cancer was back in my brain and the other tumours had grown slightly. My oral chemo had stopped being effective, which meant I would have to go back on to intravenous chemo, although apparently my hair wouldn't fall out this time. There has to be a silver lining, right?

Dr Houston didn't sugarcoat the news. I knew it was about managing the disease now, not curing it, and I didn't need any false hope. It would have been wonderful if he could have told me something good, but there was really nothing good to say.

I felt a bit numb to it all at that point. I could hear his words, but I wasn't really taking them in, just nodding in the right places and asking the right questions. Although I'm a very positive person, there's only so much you can take. The results were crushing, but what was really getting to me was that I was losing my voice and no one seemed to understand how devastating that was for me.

I wanted to know why I was losing it and if anything could be done to treat it, but Dr Houston was almost dismissive when I brought it up and insisted the scans and X-rays hadn't shown anything.

'Oh, yes, we see that voice thing and the cough a lot,' he said.

'So what is it then?' I pushed.

'It's just something that happens. Try not to worry about it. I'll speak to one of our ear, nose and throat specialists.'

I felt as if he was fobbing me off, as if to say, 'Forget it, love. This is what happens. It's going to get worse and then you're going to go.' I felt like he was giving up on me.

I felt really bloody angry. I wanted to shout, 'Fuck off! Don't give up on me. I'm not giving up on me!'

Don't get me wrong, Dr Houston had been wonderful and I was very grateful to him, but I felt like he was being glib about something that was my life; something that meant everything to me. I'd been singing since I was two years old. I know this may seem a bizarre thing to say, but the fear of losing my voice was almost greater than the fear of the cancer. Of course, if it was a toss-up between losing my voice and living, I would choose to lose my voice, but singing is in my blood and in my bones, it is part of who I am. It gives me so much pleasure. It isn't just a job.

Once we'd sorted out the dates for my treatment with Dr Houston, Steve and I left. Reality Check Number Two was being told I couldn't go to Thailand in February because he wanted to start my chemo on 15 January. On reflection, I didn't want to risk being ill so far away from home in a country where I didn't speak the language, but I was disappointed and I knew Steve and Erin would be too. The thought of being in such a gorgeous paradise, away from all the horrible realities of home, had kept us all going. I had to face up to the fact that I'd probably never make it to Thailand. But I told myself that the important thing was staying alive, and hopefully that's what the chemo would achieve.

There wasn't much to feel good about after that appointment with Dr Houston, but being the naturally optimistic soul that I am, I still managed to find a tiny sliver of positivity to cling on to. He could have told me there was nothing more he could do to contain the cancer, but he didn't. There was still a treatment plan and that was something for me to focus on. Things hadn't taken a total nosedive – OK, the cancer had grown, but it was still fairly small and it hadn't moved anywhere else.

Steve and I felt shattered, but our major concern was how and what to tell Erin. In the end, we decided to tell her that the cancer had come back and that it had grown a bit, but not to reveal that it was back in my brain. I really felt that was too much for her to deal with. She'd been so excited when I'd told her it was gone from my brain, and she'd even said to me, 'You know what, Mum? It's gone from your brain, so things might have improved again.' I didn't want to take that away from her.

I called my sisters and brothers to tell them. They were pissed off and angry, but nobody cried. I guess they may have cried on their own, but they didn't do it in front of me. I'm sure they were doing their best to stay strong and positive for my sake. I'd taught them well!

Getting the results of my scans just before Christmas was terrible timing, but we still managed to have a nice time. Maureen, Richie and Linda came to stay. The past couple of weeks had been very stressful, so it was lovely that it was just the six of us. As usual, Steve outdid himself with the food. On Christmas Eve he made fillet steak with a porcini mushroom sauce and a tarte tatin for dessert. Then on Christmas Day we had our traditional lobster starter. This year we had three live lobsters in the fridge: Curly, Larry and Mel. Steve made a tarragon and lime dressing to drizzle over them and they were delicious – sorry guys! And of course, the turkey main course was amazing as always.

There were no sad faces at Christmas. You wouldn't have had to try too hard to glimpse the sadness hiding beneath the surface, but nobody showed it. We watched loads of movies in front of the fire – *The Grinch* and *It's a Wonderful Life*, which we always cry at! I imagine it was what an old person's Christmas is like! It was totally different to our previous Christmases, which have been much boozier affairs with lots of singing around the table, but I felt totally relaxed.

Steve wouldn't let me lift a finger, but I was worried about him. He must have been knackered because he'd been doing everything – cooking, cleaning, grocery shopping, sorting out the bedrooms for my sisters and Richie, putting up the decorations. He'd even sprayed snow on all the windowpanes because he knows how much I love that. And, of course, he must have been worrying about me too, which is exhausting in itself.

My plan was to go back to panto in Eastbourne on Boxing Day, but I had to be able to talk and I still couldn't do it without coughing my head off. I could mime the songs, but I needed to project my voice on stage, particularly as I played a wicked character. If I got into a coughing fit, I wouldn't be able to stand on the stage for two minutes until it stopped. And the stress of trying not to cough was becoming too much for me.

I didn't want to ruin the production for the cast and the audience, and I knew I had to make that call to say I wasn't coming back, but I kept putting it off. Every day, I'd call Chris, the producer, and say, 'I can't come in today, but hopefully I'll be there tomorrow . . .' He was so patient and never pushed me to make a decision. But in the end I knew I had to call it a day so I rang one of my agents, Amanda, to tell her.

I was devastated about it though. In twenty years of performing in panto, I'd never taken a day off sick but, physically, I just wasn't up to it. As well as the cough and having no voice, I felt completely exhausted. I couldn't fight it any more; I had to walk away.

I had my professional pride too. I was sounding crap and I had never been crap in my life. I couldn't perform to the best of my ability, which was embarrassing, and I didn't want the cast feeling on edge all the time because of me.

Not being able to sing was killing me. I couldn't even sing for pleasure. I hadn't been able to sing 'Auld Lang Syne' at New Year and I'd always been the one to stand up at parties and sing something, usually egged on by Maureen. I'd sung Erin to sleep every single night since the day she was born and I couldn't do that any more either. It was hell and I began to get increasingly frustrated.

'I refuse to just sit around and accept that I can't sing, that I can barely speak,' I said to Steve one day. I wasn't naïve enough to believe I'd be doing any major roles on stage in the future, but I wanted a voice! No one had ever warned me that I might lose my voice. It was a cruel surprise.

But the doctors continued to be vague about it and it really pissed me off. I assumed they were too scared to tell me what was causing it and what the likely outcome would be. But I wanted to know: Will it get better? Will it get worse? Will I lose my voice totally? Is it cancer? What is it?! I was driving myself mad.

All these negative thoughts started to whirl around in my brain. I'm a huge supporter of the NHS, but I started to wonder if the doctors would listen to me more if I were paying for treatment. I began questioning everything: 'Am I not a priority any more? Would they rather deal with people who have more chance of living?' That's how I felt, which I know is terrible and not like me at all.

The two weeks following Christmas were hard and Steve and I had to dig really deep to pull ourselves out of it. Erin was in bed with the flu and I'd pulled a muscle in my shoulder, which was really painful. It was a really miserable time. And because I'd given up work, I was sitting at home all day with nothing to do except think about my treatment – or the lack of it. It had been three weeks since my appointment with Dr Houston and I hadn't been taking any medication during that time, which made me really edgy. I had an aggressive form of cancer and I couldn't help thinking it must be growing and spreading with nothing to fight it. Dr Houston had told me three weeks without chemo wouldn't do me any harm, but I felt like shit. I was short of breath and there never seemed to be a moment when I wasn't coughing. I had a few hospital appointments lined up over the next few days – I was having radiotherapy on my back to ease the pain as well as my first chemo session – so I was determined to get some answers.

The way I was feeling started to take its toll on my relationship with Steve. Usually, I'm the one to bring everybody up – I have a naturally sunny disposition and Steve doesn't – so if I'm down, we've had it. And I found those two weeks after Christmas really, really hard. I was dealing with heavy stuff so of course there were going to be times when I lost it and cried, and felt angry or just desperately sad. It was bound to happen, and it did happen during those two weeks. I wasn't crying for myself so much, but I felt sad for Steve and Erin. I'd had bad patches in the past, but this one was taking a bit longer to get to grips with. Normally I'd be over it and focusing on my treatment and feeling well again, but it just felt different this time. When I'd first been diagnosed with breast cancer, I knew I was having the breast removed and that the cancer was going with it. But, as I've said before, it's a whole different ball game when the disease has invaded your body and there is no cure. And I was feeling physically ill, too, which didn't help my mood. The first time around I hadn't felt ill – the chemo had made me tired and it was undeniably hard sometimes – but I knew it was just the drugs. Now I was lying in bed at night, unable to sleep, obsessing over every ache and pain. Were they normal aches and pains or were they to do with the cancer?

Steve and I started rowing over everything and anything – shouting and snapping at each other over stupid things that didn't matter because we were both so stressed.

Steve was really struggling, so his way of dealing with things was to focus on being practical. He massaged my bad shoulder tirelessly every night. I told him he didn't have to keep doing it because it must have been boring and his hands must have ached, but he said it made him feel useful.

He also drove down to Eastbourne to pack up all my gear from the panto because I couldn't face going back and seeing everyone.

'It'll be done then and we can start afresh,' he'd said brightly, as he was leaving that day. But when he called later to tell me he was on his way home, his mood had changed and he was upset.

'When I drove through the town there was a billboard advertising the panto with your picture on it, and it was so sad,' he told me, struggling to keep his emotions in check. 'Someone had put your stuff from the dressingroom in a nice box and that upset me, too. It's like the cancer has won this one.'

'Stop it, Steve!' I replied. 'We said we wouldn't do this. Come on! We've got to hold it together. Don't bloody cry.'

But it wasn't fair of me to react like that – he should have been able to cry if he'd wanted to. Although it was great for me to see him being so strong all the time, it wasn't good for him. He was going through hell too, and he needed to be allowed to deal with my illness in his own way, but he didn't want to bring me down. He needed someone to talk to and rant at and cry in front of. As much as I tried, though, I couldn't be Steve's shoulder to cry on because I needed him too much. I needed him to be my rock.

Linda was always trying to encourage me to see a counsellor because it had helped her a lot when she had breast cancer, but my illness had taken a different course to hers. Plus, I knew I wouldn't benefit from it – I didn't want to feel forced to talk about it and it would have felt like wallowing to me. It just wasn't my kind of thing. If I didn't want to confide in Steve, I knew I could pick up the phone and talk to one of my sisters or a friend, and I had the wonderful breast cancer nurses for support too. I had lots of options, but I did accept that side of things was harder for Steve. Generally, it's harder for men to open up to their friends and family. I suggested to him that he might benefit from seeing a counsellor and said that I'd be able to organise it through the nurses at the hospital. I was amazed when he said he'd consider it, but I wasn't sure he meant it. I hoped he did.

At the time, I wasn't that easy to live with. Everyone told me I was being so strong and called me brave all the time, but I was also bloody moody and irritable and very stressed, especially because I couldn't speak properly. My voice had become so soft, it was almost like a whisper.

Steve constantly had to ask me to repeat what I'd said because he couldn't hear me and it drove me absolutely insane. I felt disabled.

I used to get really angry and shout at him – or at least I tried to shout!

He was angry too – angry at the whole situation. One day we had a row over something silly and he said to me, 'Why don't you leave, Bernie? Why don't you just leave if you're so frustrated and stressed?'

'Don't be bloody ridiculous!' I snapped back.

We sniped at each other out of sheer frustration and I kept telling myself it was just a blip and that we'd get over it once I started my next round of chemo. The most frustrating thing of all was sitting at home without medication, imagining the tumours growing bigger inside me. To be brutally frank, it scared the shit out of me. I wanted to feel like I was doing something to get well. I wanted those chemotherapy drugs coursing through my veins. But I knew the drugs had to be ordered in specially and a treatment plan had been worked out for me, which I had to stick to. I would just have to sit tight and wait another few days.

I was concerned about how the past couple of weeks had affected Erin. She was behaving like a mini me really. I overheard her saying to her friends that I was 'living with cancer, not dying from it', which was my line! I'd said that to her lots of times to try to keep her positive.

Maybe she was in a bit of denial about my condition but, at thirteen, was that such a bad thing? I didn't want her to know every detail of what I was going through.

I wasn't going to sit her down and say to her, 'You know what, Erin, I could die,' but I think she understood that deep down.

I was glad that she still felt able to behave like a normal teenager. She still asked if her friends could come to the house for sleepovers and she wanted to go out and do things with her mates, too. But I also wanted her to know she could cry if she felt like it and not to feel worried about upsetting me.

It was tricky knowing how to get the balance right. I didn't want to upset her by talking about my illness too much, but I also wanted her to feel she could be open and honest with me about how she was feeling. I kept saying to her, 'You know you can ask me or your dad anything, or you can speak to one of your aunties.' She knew there were plenty of people around to confide in.

I could tell when she was stressed, though. Sometimes she'd behave a little selfishly and Steve would say to her, 'Look, be nice to your mum for God's sake, she's not well.'

'I know she's not well. Do you think I'm stupid?!' she would snap back.

Like Steve and me, she was just frustrated. It was a new and stressful situation for all of us; a living nightmare. Deep down, of course she was worried. One day she said to me, 'Mum, you're not going to die are you?' She'd asked me that a few times in the past and I'd always said, 'Don't be stupid!' but this time I couldn't bring myself to just say 'No.'

'We're all going to die, Erin,' I said gently.

'Arrgh, I don't like you saying that. You've never said

that before,' she replied, shaking her head. 'Why are you saying it now? Something must have changed, the cancer must be worse.'

'Well, you know it's come back and we're fighting it with chemo. We've just got to keep fighting. That's all we can do.'

I couldn't bring myself to say there was a chance it might not work. I wanted her to keep faith and carry on as normal for as long as possible. But because things had been stressful at home over the previous couple of weeks, I knew I had to keep a close eye on her.

I felt so guilty about how my illness was affecting Steve and Erin. At one point I even tried to persuade them to go to Thailand in February without me. 'Go, you'll have the holiday of a lifetime,' I said, trying my hardest to sound enthusiastic. 'It'll be lovely just the two of you. You can do some father-daughter bonding. Just think about that gorgeous swimming pool outside our room!'

Of course, neither of them wanted to leave me behind, but I went on about it so much they said they would think about it.

However, when I was sitting on my own one day, I imagined waving them both off at the airport and suddenly I didn't want them to go at all. Steve and Erin were my lifeline and the thought of them leaving sent me into a total panic. Linda would have come to stay with me, so I wouldn't have been alone, but I just couldn't bear the idea of them being so far away. I didn't say anything, though. How could I? I'd made such a song and dance about them going off and having a great time, trying to convince them I'd be fine on my own for a couple of weeks.

When Erin finally decided she didn't want to go to Thailand, Steve said to me, 'How did you really feel about us going without you?'

'Oh, God, I'm so relieved you're not going!' I blurted out, unable to hide my relief.

'You bloody idiot, Bernie! Why didn't you say something?' he said, laughing and pulling me in for a hug.

'Look, I don't want to stop you and Erin doing anything, that's why.'

I really wished I'd made it to Thailand years before. It was one of those places I'd always dreamt about and now I couldn't go. And I was pissed off about it! The moral of this story is, if you have the cash or the opportunity to do something you've always wanted to do, don't wait, just bloody do it! Don't keep saying, 'Oh, I'll do it next year,' just in case the universe has other plans for you.

At my next hospital visit in mid-January, I let out three weeks' worth of anger and frustration on my lovely breast cancer nurse Olga! I wasn't naïve enough to believe I was suddenly going to be cured of cancer – I knew all I had was treatment – but I wanted to be put in the picture about my throat and I needed to feel reassured they were still on my side and doing everything they could for me. I'm the sort of person who responds to positivity and sitting at home for weeks with nothing to work towards and no information was very hard.

'Look, Olga, I need to tell you how I feel,' I said assertively, as soon as Steve and I were seated in her office. 'This isn't your cancer and it's not his cancer,' I continued, pointing at Steve. 'It's my cancer and I want everyone to fight for me like I'm fighting for me. I know you're looking after God knows how many other patients, Olga, but I don't want to get forgotten.'

I understand the NHS is swamped with patients and stretched to breaking point when it comes to resources but, trust me, when you're the one with cancer, you want to be an important patient and you want those resources directed at you. I needed all my energy to fight the disease; I couldn't take on the hospital too. I felt I had to stamp my foot a bit to be heard and I felt a lot better after getting it off my chest.

Olga was so calm and collected – she just sat and listened and promised to see what she could do. Dr Houston was busy that day, so I didn't get to talk to him, but I managed to see Mr Kissin and I offloaded on him, too.

'There's still loads more we can do,' he said reassuringly. 'We haven't even got a whole rabbit out of the bag yet.'

It was exactly what I needed to hear. I just wanted to feel listened to; even that phrase about the rabbit gave me something to hold on to!

After I saw Olga, everything started to change. The breast cancer nurses called me at home more regularly and another doctor, Dr Saleh, really took on my case. He reminded me of a lovely grandad and on the day of my first chemo session he knew I was a bit scared, so he came to check on me.

'How are you doing, Bernie?' he asked kindly. 'I want to help you in every way I know how and to make you well and feel good again.' And I knew that he meant it.

As it turned out, my first chemo session was absolutely fine, but starting new chemotherapy drugs was always a bit daunting after the terrifying allergic reaction I'd had the very first time.

I also had to have an MRI scan to check what the cancer was doing in my brain and that was much worse than the chemo. I was drugged, so I was absolutely out of it, but I still felt really claustrophobic and panicked lying flat on my back in that narrow tube, and it was very noisy as well. I hated it.

I was told the only way to tackle the cancer in my brain was to have radiotherapy, which I found a pretty scary prospect. I got measured for a special mask, which would keep my head totally still during treatment – they didn't want to zap the good bits, after all! It meant we had to tell Erin that the cancer was back in my brain and explain the treatment because there were side effects associated with it. It can cause fits, short-term memory loss, hair loss and I would probably be incredibly tired, too.

My heart sank at the thought of giving Erin more difficult news to get her head around, but it wasn't fair to keep her in the dark – we were all in this together, which is how it should be. And I wouldn't be able to hide those kinds of side effects from her anyway.

She was shocked when we told her what the radiotherapy would entail and I admitted to her that I was scared about it, but she said, 'You're having the radiotherapy, Mum!'

'Oh really, you've decided that, have you?' I replied.

'Yes! You're having everything you need.'

Erin has never been backward at giving me a lecture or doing a bit of cheerleading to give me a boost if she thinks I need it. Like mother, like daughter, eh?

But I was worried about the hair loss thing because she'd hated it when my hair fell out during my first round of chemo, probably because it was such an obvious sign that I was sick. And let's be honest, it would be shocking and upsetting for anyone to see their mum looking like that. I completely got it. So this time I decided to deal with it differently. I was told my hair would come out in patches with radiotherapy rather than all over, so I decided to keep it long and just comb over strands of hair to hide the bald bits. And instead of bandanas, I was going to wear beanie hats. So that was my fashion and beauty regime sorted!

I was also prescribed steroids to take down the swelling in my brain, which the cancer was causing. And the steroids would also help to combat symptoms such as headaches, dizziness and fits. All of this, plus the intravenous chemo, would carry on indefinitely until it stopped working, which I hoped wouldn't be for a long time.

I realised this was a lot to take on and that it wouldn't be easy, but what choice did I have? I guess I could sit at home and cry every day and wait to die, but I didn't want to do that. I wanted to live.

The last time I'd seen Olga she'd given me a book about living with secondary breast cancer to take away and read. It had stories about people who had been living with cancer for a while and I found it really encouraging. When I'd first been diagnosed, I wanted to blank that kind of thing out. I really didn't want to know. But now my situation was different. There was no cure, so I had to just try to keep going and stay alive. These people talked about the importance of putting nice things into their lives

– holidays, experiences and social events – while they were undergoing treatment. There were women on their third round of chemo. You have to find ways of still enjoying your life when you're going through something so gruelling.

I'd come across inspiring women myself. My nephew Danny, Maureen's son, has a relative on his fiancée's side who has had cancer five times and she's beaten it every time. She's seventy, she's still here and she's really attractive and full of life. I wanted to be like her.

I had to carry on and fill my life with things other than hospital appointments – I knew I would go mad if I didn't! I promised myself that in the coming months I would plan holidays and get-togethers with friends and family – stuff to look forward to. And I was lucky to have Erin around – she still needed a social secretary to keep track of sleepovers and parties, and someone to nag her about her homework.

I can't explain how I was still able to find hope in such a difficult situation. It wasn't denial, but I never wanted my oncologist to say to me, 'I'm sorry, there's no hope for you.' I didn't want to know that, even if it was the truth, because I wanted to carry on for as long as I could, with hope and with fun, and that was my choice.

16
MAKING PLANS

....

One afternoon at the end of January 2013, I was lying on the sofa in front of the fire, lazily flicking through the TV channels when I began thinking of a holiday we'd had in Rome the year before for Steve's fiftieth birthday. It was February 2012, two months before I found out the cancer had returned, and we were happy and carefree.

I'd rented a big beautiful apartment with full-length windows that looked on to the famous Piazza Navona. Erin and Linda were with us, and my brother Brian and his wife Annie.

On one of the evenings we decided to stay in and Steve cooked us a fabulous meal, and we drank loads of lovely Italian wine. It wasn't long before Linda and Brian started nagging me to sing.

'Sing out of the window, Bernie,' said Linda.

'Get lost! You're mad,' I replied, laughing.

'Go on, Bernie, give them some soprano out the window. Do something from *Popstar to Operastar*,' said Brian.

I was a bit drunk, so I said, 'Oh, Christ, go on then.'

I walked over to the window and started to sing 'Parla

Più Piano' from *The Godfather*, which everyone had loved when I'd performed it on the show.

The piazza was quiet, but there were about six people walking past and when they heard me sing they stopped and I saw one of them point up to my window. They all stood still, listening, and when I'd finished they broke into a round of applause and started shouting, '*Bravo! Encore! Encore!*'

I was giggling like a naughty schoolgirl and Brian was saying, 'Do it again. Do it again!' while Annie got her phone out, ready to film it so she could show Maureen when she got home.

So I did it again and by this time there were about two hundred people in the piazza, staring up at the window and calling their friends over to listen. They all cheered and clapped at the end, and I actually felt quite overcome with emotion. 'That was amazing, Mum,' Erin said, immediately Facebooking all her friends with the clip.

Being able to sing like that is truly wonderful. I'd only done it for a laugh that night, but it gave me a feeling of pure joy. Sadly, I would never be able to do anything like that again. I knew that for sure now.

Stephen Houston had referred me to a couple of cancer experts who specialise in the head and neck area, and I'd been back to the Royal Surrey to see them. I had another camera down my throat and this time I was left in no doubt of the results.

The consultant Dr Katie Wood told me straight away I had vocal paralysis, which was the result of tumours around my sternum pressing on my left vocal cord. An operation was possible, but it would be an extremely dangerous procedure and could even prove fatal. It was not something they generally recommend.

'Sod it,' I thought. 'I'm trying to stay alive here. I'm not risking surgery that could kill me!'

I had to steel myself for what I was about to say next.

'Let's just get this out in the open and establish it as fact now – will I ever sing again?' I asked, dreading her reply.

'No, I don't think you will,' she said. 'Because one of your vocal cords is paralysed, you simply wouldn't have the power.'

God, I had to swallow so hard to get rid of the lump in my throat. I could easily have lost it, sitting there in her consulting room, but I hate crying in front of people, so I did my best to hold it together. When I got home later that day, though, I let the floodgates open. I cried and cried. For me, it was a devastating loss. I suppose deep down I already knew I would never sing again, but to have it confirmed was truly heartbreaking. In the context of how ill I was, some people might not understand why not being able to sing was so upsetting. Well, I'd been singing on stage since the age of two when my first performance of 'Show Me the Way to Go Home' won me a gold watch in that talent competition at the end of Blackpool pier. Singing had been my life for fifty years and being told I'd never do it again not only meant the end of my career, it meant the end of that part of me. In terms of what the cancer did to my body, taking away my voice was the cruellest part.

There was a little good news, though. Believe it or not, I managed to find some. I was told I could have injections in my throat to bolster my vocal cord and I was also referred to a speech therapist. I felt a million times better after I'd seen her. At my first appointment she told me my vocal cords had 'good closure', which was an encouraging sign. 'Most people at your stage who come to me have no closure at all,' she said.

I was given vocal exercises and other exercises like yawning to help relax the muscles in my throat. She also tried to massage my larynx, but it was too painful and I was sick, so we shelved that one for another time.

I had ten appointments booked and to me that felt like working. I'd go so far as to say it was fun. Hey, in my situation you have to get it where you can! Being a singer I understood the voice and I wanted to get stuck in. Improving my speech was something I could focus on over the coming weeks, something to aim for.

I was being as positive as I could, but there was no denying the fact the tide had turned. The news was bad, I had deteriorated and it was starting to affect me emotionally as well as physically. I was feeling unwell and the side effects of the cancer were now worse than the chemo. Previously, it had been the drugs making me feel crappy, not the disease. Sometimes, when I was sitting in that waiting-room at the Royal Surrey, I wanted to scream the place down. I was so sick of sitting there, waiting to be given bad news.

It was hard and I can't say there were many light moments at the beginning of 2013. The first happy time in weeks was when Brian and Annie came to stay for a couple of nights. Steve and I had been feeling so down and we really, really needed them – they have a brilliant sense of fun and make us laugh, and they think we're hilarious as a couple, too! We have always got along really well as a foursome and Steve and I could be ourselves in front of them.

They turned up on a Friday night and transformed the atmosphere completely. Steve cooked a gorgeous casserole and we had lots of red wine. I coughed my head off and didn't care. I swore, drank, laughed and stayed up late! It was marvellous. I felt like a normal person again.

My friend Rick – a music director – also came to stay for a night. He was working on *Boogie Nights* with my nephew Shane Jnr, Coleen's eldest son. And Linda popped down too, on her way to visit her step-granddaughter, who was expecting her first baby. It was so good to see everyone – it cheered me up.

And although I wouldn't exactly call it a light moment, I also opened a new surgical breast care unit at the Royal Surrey with Mark Kissin, and it was nice to see him too, especially in a situation where he wasn't giving me terrible news!

At home, though, when it was just the three of us, it could be tough. It was very hard for Steve – he was scared and I knew he couldn't bear to imagine a life without me. There must have been so many things he wanted to get off his chest, things he didn't feel able to say to me. I tried again to get him to see a counsellor, but he insisted he only wanted to talk to me.

We'd always been such a close couple. We did everything together, which I know sounds a bit pathetic, but it's true. We've always been each other's best mate and there has never been any pretence between us. We'd far rather spend time together than have girly weekends or lads' holidays.

He has devoted his life to Erin and me, and he's an amazing husband and father. He's a bloody saint in fact! Very few men would have given up their career to stay at home to support their wife and bring up their child, but he did. He's an amazing drummer, but I earned more money than he did, so the sensible thing to do was for him to stay at home while I went out to work. He just got on with it and never complained.

But because our little family unit had always been so tight, I completely understood why he didn't feel comfortable confiding in other people, even though I thought it would help him. And, in all honesty, I couldn't force him to do something I had no intention of doing myself. As I've said before, counselling wasn't for me. I didn't want a stranger's pity or someone trying to tell me how to deal with an illness that I'd been living with every day. But I was still able to ask for help in my own way. My breast care nurse Olga was amazing and I knew I had access to community care workers, even at weekends, if I had questions or a crisis of tears. That was reassuring.

Steve and I had stopped arguing over silly things, which meant it was a lot calmer at home. The stress we'd both been feeling had been overtaken by fear, though. Let's be honest, it's frightening when your brain gets involved and it's terrible to see someone you love get fitted for a scary-looking Perspex mask so they can be blasted with gamma rays. It was just very sad for all of us.

I tried to get Steve to look on the bright side of radiotherapy – if there is such a thing – in that it was something that could make me feel well again. It was the only option we had, so we had to go for it. It meant we were still moving forward. And who was to say the treatment wouldn't make things better? My last lot of drugs had been really effective at first. All I could do was hope that I'd have the same luck this time around.

My attitude was to take every bit of good news – however small – and focus on it to the exclusion of everything else. I tried to approach every day as a new beginning and think, 'Right, what's next? What do we have to do now?' I couldn't sit around thinking, 'I'm going to die.' It's torture living with the fact you have an incurable disease, but at least you have time and I was determined to buy myself as much time as possible.

Erin had started having a bit of a bad time, which worried me. I think the change in her mood was partly down to the fact that my symptoms were becoming more obvious. I couldn't speak properly, I'd started slurring my words, I'd stopped singing, I needed to rest more and now the vision in my left eye was blurred, too. All those changes were happening right in front of her.

Everyone at her school was superb. Steve and I spoke to a couple of her teachers and explained that I was having more treatment. They offered Erin counselling and time off whenever she needed it, and gave her a pass for the counselling room so she could leave class whenever she wanted to. And she'd obviously been talking about what was happening at home. When Steve spoke to the school counsellor, she told him that Erin had had a bit of a wobble and she'd come down to the counselling room to have a chat with her.

But I was pleased she felt able to confide in other people. She probably had tons of questions she didn't want to ask me, like 'Will my mum go nuts?' because the cancer was in my brain.

One afternoon she came home from school and Steve said to her, 'Are you angry with us, Erin?'

'Yeah, I am actually,' she replied softly.

'We totally understand,' Steve continued. 'We're angry, too, and we don't know how to deal with it either. But we're adults and you're a kid, so it's extra hard for you.'

Then she asked me again if I was going to die. She'd been asking me that a lot lately. I think she was beginning to doubt my positive attitude.

'Everything I've told you is the truth,' I said. 'The cancer isn't curable. It's never going to go away. All they can do is try to keep me alive with drugs and radiotherapy. But none of my doctors has ever said to me it's not treatable. None of them has ever said I'm dying.'

That was all true, but it must have been really hard for Erin to see me so ill. She'd known me as this fun-loving energetic person and now the disease was turning me into someone she didn't recognise. Which is why I was determined to keep everything else in her life as familiar as possible. Because I wasn't going to be able to work in the coming year, we should have put our house in Weybridge up for sale and moved to St Anne's or Blackpool to be mortgage free, but I didn't want to take Erin out of school or away from her friends. She'd lived in Weybridge her entire life and I wanted her to have a sense of stability and continuity. I'd never had that as a child because I was always on the road performing with The Nolans, so I loved the fact that Erin had grown up in one place. I liked to imagine her when she was older, meeting up with her friends at the local cafés and bars, and feeling she was part of a community. I decided that if it came down to it, we could always rent our house and get a smaller place – whatever it took so she could stay in the area. It was all about Erin.

Erin and I aren't like most mums and daughters in that we don't shop together and do girly things – neither of us is very girly! She prefers her Xbox to most things! She always asks me to play it with her, but I'm crap and she ends up shouting, 'You're rubbish, Mum, get off!'

Like most teens she's also into Facebook and her gang of friends, and most of the time Steve and I are just 'boring' and 'don't know what we're talking about'. She's thirteen – it's completely normal! I love that about her.

I didn't want Erin to be sitting on the sofa at home with me all the time feeling upset. Steve and I were at the raw end of this shitty disease. We had to deal with it, but she could be shielded from it to some extent. I told myself she would deal with things when the time came, although I couldn't bear to even go there in my head. It just didn't bear thinking about. In the meantime, I wanted her to go out and have fun and do all the things she did before I became ill.

Like me, Erin loves to travel, so I decided my mission for 2013 would be to plan lots of trips. It was important to feel we had some good things to look forward to, particularly as we'd missed out on our family holiday to Thailand. So I set about writing a list of must-do dream holidays for the three of us that didn't involve a twelve-hour flight!

Top of the list was Venice. I'd wanted to take her there for ages, so she could see where Steve had asked me to marry him. And I could tell her the story again of how he couldn't find the Rialto Bridge where he'd planned to propose and how we'd nearly missed our ship!

I'd already organised a week in Blackpool in February to see my family and planned a big celebration meal for Steve's fifty-first birthday, which was on 19 February. The Pleasure Beach may not be quite as exotic as our luxury Thai resort, where he should have been spending his birthday, but we'd have fun nonetheless! Brian said he'd put us up (including our dog Dexter!), Coleen was coming over from Cheshire and even Anne texted to say she was really looking forward to seeing me. It would be good to get everyone together.

The argument we'd had with Anne and Denise over the reunion tour was still there, lurking in the background, but it felt to me as if my illness had brought the three of us closer again. After I was diagnosed with cancer they stopped mentioning the tour. Instead they started texting to see how I was and to say they loved me. To coin a corny phrase, maybe they just realised that life's too short to drag things on. I know that's how I felt.

I was hoping my illness would help to reunite all of my sisters, but I think for Linda, and Coleen especially, too much water has gone under the bridge. The row over the tour was awful – I'll never get over Anne being left out, but some vile things were said.

But from where I stand – as someone with incurable

cancer – I can't fathom why they are still not talking to each other, and I kind of feel annoyed with all of them. It's not as if someone was murdered! But at the same time, I would never want to put pressure on any of them – they have to make their own choices in life and some things are very hard to forgive.

The whole situation makes me feel incredibly sad, but if my sisters are going to start talking again, I realise they have to do it because they want to and not because I have cancer!

Next on my list of Places To Go was Mijas in Spain, where I'd spent lots of lovely holidays with Steve and Erin. My cousin Allan Foran was celebrating his sixtieth birthday out there in March with his wife Angie and lots of their mates, so we were going too, and so were Brian and Annie. I'd managed to get travel insurance so I booked our flights – I just had to cross my fingers I'd be well enough to fly when the time came and that my doctors would let me get on the plane! I figured it was a short flight and I'd only be away for a week. And maybe one of the consultants could give me a letter explaining my condition like they did when I went to Maureen's wedding in Spain during my first lot of chemo. I figured things would be clearer once I'd started the radiotherapy.

After Mijas I wanted to go on another road trip around England, visiting friends and relatives like we'd done the summer after I'd been diagnosed with breast cancer. There's nowhere on earth more beautiful when the sun is shining. And it would be an opportunity to reconnect with people we hadn't seen in a while.

Coleen had also bought a weekend in a gorgeous cottage

in the Lake District at a charity event and she'd given it to me as a pressie. So that was our trip for May sorted! I don't get to see Coleen as much as Linda and Maureen because she's always so busy with work and with her own family, but she calls or texts practically every day to see how I am, and we always manage to have a laugh.

Also on my list was booking a minibreak for the 'Weybridge Eight' – that's Steve, Erin, Linda, Brian, Annie, Maureen, Richie and me. We started going away together after I won a trip to a hotel in Shropshire at a charity auction. We had a ball for three days and after that it became a regular thing. For this year's trip I wanted to go to the Cotswolds and I found a picture-perfect English cottage with a big log fire, surrounded by cute villages and beautiful countryside – and with a golf course nearby for the boys!

OK, maybe the next two on my list were pipe dreams, but I wanted to go to New York with Steve and Erin in the summer and I also had this fantasy about spending next Christmas in an Alpine chalet surrounded by snow-capped mountains. I imagined the three of us going for sleigh rides and falling out of toboggans, and racing in from the cold to a cosy lounge with a crackling fire and some of my favourite music on the stereo – Sinatra, Tony Bennett, Michael Bublé, James Taylor and Stephen Bishop. If radiotherapy and more chemo could help me to achieve those dreams, then bring it on.

I was absolutely determined to keep going, to keep fighting. Steve once told me I could be that 'miracle girl' who beat the odds and defied the doctors' predictions, and I'd always held on to that thought. Why shouldn't I be that girl? I love my life and my family too much to think any other way. If there was even the slightest chance that treatment could help me to see the milestones in Erin's life, I was going to take it.

I have always been someone who has lived life to the full and there are still so many things I want to do. What really pisses me off about dying is the thought that I'm going to miss everything. I feel jealous when I think about all the parties and Christmases everyone's going to have without me. It's just doesn't seem right – I've always been the party animal! So I'm going to enjoy the life I have for as long as I possibly can.

A FINAL WORD:
COUNTING MY BLESSINGS

....

I've been counting my blessings, which might seem an odd thing to do, considering I have cancer that can't be cured. But I wouldn't be Bernie if I couldn't find that glimmer of light in the dark. There's no question that writing this book has made me confront the cold reality of my current situation, but it's also made me realise what a full and wonderful life I've had, and how much I still have to be grateful for.

Growing up as one of eight children in a big, chaotic, loving Irish family has blessed me with such a strong sense of love and security, and I carry that with me every day. I'm thankful for my sisters and my lovely brothers, Tommy and Brian – I can't quite believe I chose to live in Surrey while they all stayed in Blackpool.

Steve is the love of my life. I don't know what I did to deserve him, but my life has been made very special by knowing him. He makes sacrifices for me daily, he's always by my side and he's an amazing dad to Erin. I love the fact he has strong opinions and isn't afraid to speak his mind, and I feel so lucky I'm with a man who sticks to what he believes in no matter what.

I've grown up a lot since meeting Steve and I've learnt so much through him – to rely on myself before anyone else, to be true to who I really am and to be honest with other people.

Like most couples, we've had our differences – we're both very strong willed – but there has always been mutual respect and an abundance of love. Every day since meeting Steve I have felt so cherished and protected, and I count my blessings that he's been a part of my life.

Like my mum always said, Erin is a blessing from God. I loved her from the first moment I held her in my arms, unconditionally and everlastingly. She changed my life. I know I could kill for her, I would die for her, I would do anything on earth for her. She is so brave and mature, and has such kindness for everyone. She will be such a fabulous woman. It's hard to find words that truly describe how she makes me feel every day – proud, lucky, blessed. She is my angel.

My life has also been blessed by music. I've been singing professionally for fifty years and now my voice has been taken away, I feel so glad I got the chance to make my solo album. If anyone wants to play something of mine when I'm gone, that's what to play. I'm grateful Erin will have it to keep her company, too. And it has the beautiful song Steve wrote for Kate, the daughter we were blessed with first, who sadly didn't get to see any of this life. In the album sleeve I wrote: 'Whenever I've been happy, music has helped me celebrate. When I've been sad, it's been a friend. Music has never let me down.' And, over the past three years, those words have never had more poignancy.

So I haven't done too badly, have I? I've had a wonderful child, a great husband, a lovely home, a fantastic family, beautiful friends and a career that's lasted half a century. And I've had lots of fun and laughter along the way.

Bernie Nolan, January 2013

EPILOGUE

....

From Bernie's husband Steve Doneathy

Throughout her illness Bernie has never stopped planning for the future – it's her way of sticking two fingers up to the cancer. Determined as ever to keep looking forward with optimism, she booked loads of holidays for 2013. I didn't know if we'd make one of them or all of them, but I knew it was important for Bernie to put those dates in her diary. She had to have things to aim for.

She was really excited about going to Blackpool to see her family during Erin's half term week in February but, sadly, it didn't turn out to be the relaxing break we'd hoped for.

Things got off to a good start – we drove up north on Sunday 17th in our new BMW 4x4, which Bernie loved, and she kept remarking how easy it made the journey. At this point we didn't know if the radiotherapy on her brain was having any effect, but her hair had started to fall out as a result of the treatment.

My 51st birthday was on Tuesday 19th and, without me knowing, Bernie had booked a restaurant for a celebration meal and invited loads of friends and family, including my brother who I hadn't seen in four years. She'd really gone to town and it was really special.

But on our way into the restaurant that night she stumbled on the stairs and said, 'That's odd, my legs feel really weak and unsteady'. I was a bit worried, but once we were sat at the table, she seemed fine. She was quieter than usual, but we had a great night before heading back to my brother-in-law Brian's house where we were staying.

For the next three days we had a pretty quiet time, then on Friday evening Bernie was poorly. She had a very restless night's sleep and her breathing was shallow, so I took her to hospital first thing the following morning. She had a chest x-ray, which was fine, and they checked her SATS (oxygen levels in the blood), which were good at 96% (normal levels range between 90% and 100%). So we were told she could go home and advised not to overdo things.

Linda was having a birthday party at a restaurant that night. I told Bernie we didn't have to go, but she insisted on being there for Linda, so we went along but left about 10.30pm.

She slept OK that night, which I was relieved about because the plan was to drive back home the next day – it was the end of half term and Erin was due back at school on the Monday. So on the Sunday afternoon I went out for a quick pint with my brothers-in-law to say goodbye and while I was there I got a phone call from Bernie's cousin Alan asking me to come home because she wanted to be taken to the hospital. When I got back to Brian's Bernie was having a coughing fit that wouldn't stop and I was really quite worried, so we went back to hospital and they admitted her. This time her SATS were down to 78%, which is very low, and she was so weary she could barely lift her head. She simply wasn't getting enough oxygen into her body. The doctors started treating her with oxygen, morphine and methadone, and decided to keep her in for more tests.

I went back to Brian's that night, but the next day when I went to visit Bernie she said, 'Please don't leave me alone tonight, Steve, I'm always so scared in the night'. So that evening and the one after that, I slept in the chair by her bed.

The doctors still hadn't come back with anything concrete about what was going on and why she'd suddenly taken a turn for the worse. On Tuesday morning she looked so poorly I really didn't think she'd make it to the weekend. I remember taking her hand in mine and when I looked down I saw her fingers were blue. At that moment a breast care nurse came into the room and motioned for me follow her outside into the corridor.

'How are you doing?' she asked.

'Well, you tell me,' I replied. At this point I just wanted answers.

'Well, we need to have a conversation,' she said, leading me into a private office.

Once we'd sat down she said, 'We're looking at the end of life here Mr Doneathy'.

'Are you sure?' was all I could say because I was beginning to lose it and could feel the tears welling up. Of course I knew how ill Bernie was, but it just seemed amazing to me that just a few days before she'd been more or less her normal self.

After I'd cried for a bit, the nurse said, 'Would you like me to tell Bernie?'

At first I panicked and said 'Yes', but once I'd had a moment to think about it I said, 'Actually, no, I'll tell her'. But I had no idea what to say or how to say it.

'Be guided by Bernie,' advised the nurse, who offered to come with me for support.

So the two of us went back into Bernie's room and I sat on the edge of her bed. Taking hold of her hand, I said gently, 'Look, I've just been talking to the nurse and you're very, very poorly darling, and it's not good'.

I knew when I'd said those words to Bernie, she'd ask me straightaway if she was going to die and she did.

'Am I going to die?'

'Yes, darling.'

She was so weak, she didn't react too much, but I could see in her eyes an acknowledgement that the day she'd been dreading had finally arrived. But it wasn't a look of acceptance or resignation, it was almost a look of resentment, then she just shrugged her shoulders and said, 'Fuck'.

The next few minutes are a bit of a blur. There was lot of crying, mostly by me. Bernie seemed more angry than anything else.

'Would you like some time alone?' asked the nurse, so we both said yes, and when she left, we just held each other and said how much we loved each other. We knew Erin was coming in for a visit with Linda that afternoon and we wanted it to be just the two of us who broke the news, so I texted Linda and asked her to let me know when she'd arrived at the hospital.

When they got to the hospital I went outside to meet

Erin and bring her in, and I think at that point she realised things had changed. When we got to Bernie's room, I said to Erin, 'Your mam's very poorly and it's not good'.

Just like Bernie, she immediately said, 'Are you going to die, Mum?' and Bernie said 'Yes'.

Erin started crying and Bernie was trying to comfort her, saying, 'Don't worry, darling, you and your dad will be fine'.

'I don't care, I want you,' was all Erin said.

It was terrible and heartbreaking, and the three of us just sat there, sobbing for about 15 minutes as the news started to sink in. We'd always been upfront with Erin about Bernie's condition, but we'd made a conscious decision not to say those words – that her mum was going to die – until we actually had to. We'd always believed in being positive and giving her hope, and up until that point we really didn't know how long Bernie had – no one knew, not even her doctors.

Once we'd told Erin, I brought Linda into the room and we told her, and she managed to keep it together really well. She hugged us, then left the room quite quickly, probably to have a cry on her own.

It wasn't long before the doctors came round and suggested moving Bernie to a hospice. That's when it started to feel real and, that night, once Linda had taken Erin home, Bernie decided to plan her funeral. She chose the music she wanted, who she wanted travelling in what cars, the flowers, the order of service and where she wanted to be buried – in Blackpool with our stillborn daughter Kate.

She also found a poem she wanted me to read and I

found an Emily Dickinson poem I liked, which we thought Erin might like to read.

When Erin came to visit the next morning, one of the first things she said was, 'You should probably plan your funeral, Mum, because you'll want it the way *you* want it, won't you?'

'We've already done that, darling,' I said, then I showed her the poem on my iPhone that we wanted her to read.

'Do you want to have a look at it first and see how you feel?' I asked, handing her the phone.

She started reading it and she did it beautifully, whereas I couldn't make it past the first verse of my poem without losing it.

'What you need to do, Dad, is not think about Mum when you're reading it, just look at the words and focus on them. They're just words.'

We moved to the hospice on Wednesday 27th and Bernie was given a nice big room with two spare beds, which meant I would be able to stay with her. The next day I got a call from Olga, Bernie's breast care nurse at the Royal Surrey.

'How are you all doing?' she asked.

'Well, terrible,' I replied.

'When you get back down here Dr Houston wants to see Bernie.'

I was confused – we'd been told Bernie wasn't well enough to make the journey home. Had the hospice not told Bernie's oncologist it was an end of life situation?

'We're not coming back, Olga. We're in a hospice,' I explained. 'If you're not aware of that, there's a communication problem and Dr Houston needs to speak to the hospice now. If there's a possibility Bernie can be helped, you need to get hold of him now.'

When I said goodbye to Olga, I tracked down one of Bernie's doctors at the hospice and told him that her oncologist in London needed to know the situation. While all this was going on Bernie had actually rallied and, when I got back to her room she was looking a little better. The doctor I'd spoken to came to check on her and said he'd spoken to Dr Houston.

'I don't think this is an end of life situation because you look too well,' he said to Bernie, whose colour was improving with each passing minute. 'We don't think your condition is a result of the progression of the cancer, we think it's something else, so we're going to get a CT scan of your lungs to see what's going on.'

He went on to explain that he thought Bernie might have a pulmonary embolism (blood clot) in her lung, which is common in patients with lung cancer and would account for her very sudden deterioration. And, although it was life threatening, it was treatable. We couldn't help rejoicing at that news! We thought we'd reached the point of no return, but here we were being thrown a line.

I think because Bernie looked so terrible when she turned up at the hospital in Blackpool, they assumed it was down to a progression of the cancer. They weren't familiar with her case and hadn't seen her the previous week, but if she'd gone to the Royal Surrey looking so awful, they would immediately have known to look for something else because they'd been seeing her regularly. Crucially, Bernie had also missed out on a scan at the hospital in Blackpool. After being told it was an end of life situation, she didn't want to go ahead with it, but it would have explained what the problem was.

The CT scan of Bernie's lungs was scheduled for the following Monday, 4th March, and we were told we'd get the results on Tuesday, which meant we had four days to wait before finding out anything more. Luckily, our friends and family came to visit every day – Brian even brought our dog Dexter – so the room was always packed with visitors. It was amazing and it helped get us through the weekend.

It sounds crazy, but we were actually hoping Bernie did have a blood clot because we knew that could be treated. But the scan showed she had lymphangitis, a condition caused by cancer spreading to the lymph vessels of the lungs that resulted in inflammation and made it hard for her to get a full breath.

We were told it was treatable with steroids, but not for long, which was a blow. We'd been given hope against all the odds, only for it to be snatched away just a few days later. I'm still not sure what's harder to cope with – being told you're not going to make the weekend or that you could live for another couple of months.

The doctors had already been treating Bernie with steroids, along with blood thinning medication, methadone, morphine and paracetamol, which is why she'd rallied and was getting stronger.

It was then decided that Bernie should have a CT scan of her brain to find out if the radiotherapy was working. If it hadn't worked, Dr Houston wasn't willing to give her any more chemotherapy – it would be pointless as there were no chemotherapies left for Bernie that crossed the blood brain barrier. That floored us because we both knew in our hearts that the radiotherapy hadn't worked. Bernie's speech was slurred and her vision blurred, so we didn't have a lot of hope.

The results of the brain scan came back pretty quickly and we were told the radiotherapy hadn't worked, although the steroids were keeping the swelling at bay. So that was that. We were back to where we started and still had no idea how long Bernie had left.

Although the latest news was devastating, we didn't discuss her funeral again. She was looking a bit better every day, so I started taking her into the garden to get some fresh air. It's strange, because no matter how bad your situation is, it becomes your normality after a while. Every day we'd wake at 6am for meds, put the TV on, then breakfast would arrive at 8am and we'd eat it in our little armchairs. I'd get Bernie into the shower, then we'd sit back in our armchairs and watch more TV – I've never seen as many episodes of *Come Dine With Me* in my life! Then it was time for lunch and after that people would come by to visit, and by 9pm we'd be alone again. At night I'd rearrange the beds next to each other so we could hold hands while we watched TV and that was our routine every day for about a week and a half.

Erin had been off school all this time. Her teachers were brilliant and told me not to worry because she's bright and would catch up, but we didn't know how long Bernie had left. The hospice was a good place to be in that Bernie was getting real rest and the right treatment, but once she was stronger, we started questioning how long we could live like that, just sitting there, accepting her fate and waiting for her to deteriorate.

Bernie had always been determined to live as close to a normal life as possible and this was nowhere near normal. So we discussed going back to Weybridge with the family. They didn't think it was a good idea at first because we wouldn't have their support, but it was what we wanted. We wanted to be at home and for Erin to go back to school. Bernie could sit in her own armchair and I'd cook for her.

I remember when Bernie was told she'd be staying in Blackpool, one of the first things she said was, 'I'm never going to see my home again. I'm never going back to my house and I only left for six days'. She couldn't believe it and I couldn't believe that I'd have to make the trip home without her, so the idea of getting back to Weybridge was a little light at the end of the tunnel. It was something to aim for, which energised both of us.

The doctors agreed Bernie was well enough to make the trip, so I asked my friend Duncan to organise getting our house fitted with equipment, including a hand rail in the shower and a lift for the stairs. He called me back when he got to the house.

'Are you sitting down?' he asked.

'Yeah, why?'

'You've been burgled.'

Duncan had only managed to have a quick look around the house before the police showed up, but he told me the TV had gone and drawers in the kitchen and lounge were open and stuff was strewn all over the place.

When I went back into Bernie's room, she knew instantly that something was wrong and she's not the kind of girl you withhold information from – she simply won't have it!

'Tell me what's the matter,' she said.

'Duncan says we've been burgled.'

'Fuck. Unbelievable. What have they taken?'

'Not sure yet, but the TV is gone.'

'So what, it's just a TV.

When the police allowed Duncan upstairs, he discovered the burglars had been through Bernie's jewellery box and Erin's, too, and everything had gone. And there were clothes all over the floor. Duncan said he'd tidy up for us, so we put it to the back of our minds. There was nothing we could do about it and we had more important things to think about.

The hospice arranged an ambulance to take us back to Weybridge on Wednesday 20 March. We set off from Blackpool at 10am and were back home by 3pm. I didn't know what to expect when we got to the house, but I noticed straight away that Bernie's car had been stolen, which Duncan hadn't realised was in the driveway. It was a 10-year-old convertible Saab, but Bernie loved it.

We hadn't been home long when Duncan called.

'Look, there's something else I didn't want to tell you when you were in Blackpool,' he began. 'I know you have a little box in the front room where you keep Kate's things. They'd smashed the lock open and tipped it out on to the floor. I put it all back, but I don't know if anything was taken.'

When I put the phone down, I went into the lounge and opened up the box, and started looking through the sympathy cards. The photos of Kate were still there and

I found her little hospital bracelet, which really broke my heart. Erin came into the room to find me crying. We'd never let her see those photos because we felt they'd be too distressing for her.

'Can I see them Dad?' she asked.

'No, darling, I don't want you to,' I replied and she just hugged me.

I then had to tell Bernie.

'Is there anything missing from the box?' she asked.

'No.'

She was relieved and we hugged each other tightly.

Now we're settled back at home, we wake up at 7am every morning and I get Bernie her meds, then I organise Erin for school. I spend the day at home, cooking for Bernie and giving her meds every four hours.

It's worrying that she's so tired – she seems as tired as she was when she was admitted to the hospital in Blackpool. But we're both pleased we took the positive step to come home and be in charge of our own lives. At least we feel in control of some things.

And Bernie's fighting spirit is still there. One day we had someone come to check on us and this woman looked so sad with her head to one side and a 'poor you' expression in her eyes. She was almost reveling in Bernie's tragedy. And as poorly as Bernie was, I could see this was pissing her off!

I had to stand up and say, 'Thank you. Thanks for all your help. We'll be in touch if we need anything' and usher her out of the door.

'Don't ever let that woman in my house again, she's making me miserable!' said Bernie after the woman left.

It was great to see that little spark of feistiness from her. However ill she feels she won't have any of that nonsense!

We're not stupid, we know the situation is grim – we don't need reminding. But the district nurses who come in every day have been wonderful and treat Bernie like a young vibrant woman, not as someone to be pitied.

This week, we also had a bit of very unexpected good news that's lifted our spirits. A couple of days ago, Bernie's oncologist Dr Houston checked the scan from Blackpool and told us that, contrary to the information we'd been given, the cancer in her brain had actually shrunk. So after running some blood tests, which were also good, he wrote to an oncologist in Portsmouth, requesting that Bernie be put on a trial drug called TDM1, which could prolong her life.

She was of course delighted and is as determined as ever to keep fighting. 'Who says give up? NEVER give up!' she said to me the day Dr Houston broke the news.

So that's where we are. We're at home and we're doing our best. Despite everything, Bernie still stops to smell the roses and appreciate life. Some flowers arrived for her the other day and she said, 'Look, Steve, they're so beautiful'.

I'm very proud of her. I always have been. The truth is, honestly from the heart, she's inspired me every day since I met her and led me to do things I would never have done.

The way she's coped with her illness is awe-inspiring and I know the disease will never beat Bernie's spirit because she is so strong.

April 2013

August 2013

....

As July began, life for us continued in much the same way. Bernie remained positive and we took everything one day at a time.

The family had planned to visit the weekend of the 29th June, and it was a boost for Bernie to see everyone again. The weekend was fun – I did a barbecue and we all sat and talked long into the night, just like old times.

They were all due to leave on the Sunday but I asked them to stay a little longer because unbeknownst to Bernie, a lot of the cast from *Chicago* were going to drop in for a surprise visit. When they arrived I showed them into the back room where Bernie was sitting and they entered the little room singing 'Razzle Dazzle' from the show. Bernie's face lit up – she has always loved surprises. The cast stayed for about two hours, talking and singing songs. It was a wonderful end to a lovely weekend.

When everyone had left Bernie was very tired and we had an early night. The next day we got up as usual to face the day ahead, but it was obvious to me that Bernie was exhausted. I tried to convince myself that it was just the activity at the weekend that had tired her out, but as the day wore on it became apparent that it was more than that. By the end of the day she had slept more than usual and we had another early night.

The next morning (Tuesday) Bernie was even more tired and I knew things were taking a turn for the worse. I called everyone and told them that they should come back as soon as possible to see her, as I didn't think she had long left. They all said they were coming immediately. I called the doctor and he said he didn't think she had long. Everyone arrived later that day, by which time Bernie had become very weak. She stayed in bed and I called everyone in one at a time to have their last moments with her.

Later when the family were all together in the bedroom, she looked up to me and said very quietly, 'I love you so much'. I sobbed – I think I knew then that it would be the last time I heard her say that.

I stayed with Bernie the entire time, and the whole family slept at the house on sofas and inflatable beds. By the Tuesday evening she was extremely weak. I lay with her and sang songs we loved to her, and I could see a faint smile come to her face.

After a while I realised I should call everyone up to the room, since it was clear to me that Bernie was aware of the presence of people. Although by now she was too weak to even open her eyes, I knew it would make her happy to hear the chatter of her loved ones. The girls sang to her in the harmonies they'd all sang together for all those years, and again we talked into the night.

The next morning I woke up and quickly looked over to Bernie. She was still with me, but her breathing was now very shallow. Again I called everyone to the bedroom and we all stayed with her, talking and crying, and sharing memories of happier times.

Bernie passed away at 10.05am on the 4 July 2013. She was surrounded by everyone she loved, with Erin and I cradling her, stroking her hair, and telling her how much we loved her.

I still can't believe she's gone. Some days it feels as though the last 20 years have been a wonderful dream, but now I've woken up. All I want to do is go back to sleep to return to my dream.

I miss her every minute of every day and I know I'll never get over it. She was the love of my life.

Bernie's funeral was held in Blackpool with 700 friends and family filling the Grand Theatre. The streets were lined with hundreds and hundreds of people all applauding as we drove slowly through the town. Blackpool came to a standstill that day; it was as wonderful as such a sad day could be.

Erin read 'Do Not Stand at My Grave and Weep' by Mary Elizabeth Fry. She showed such poise and maturity, I know her mum would have been so proud.

I read my eulogy to Bernie, and I have decided to include it here:

Firstly, thanks to everyone for coming here for Bernie today.

Bernie loved all her friends and family, and nothing made her happier than a big get-together.

I don't have to tell anyone here or anyone who met Bernie – however briefly – how amazing and beautiful she was. Incapable of hatred, envy, bitterness or greed, she was the most honest and loyal person I've ever known, in every way.

Bernie radiated love, life and happiness. She showed me what true love was and it was beautiful. Every day was an adventure and I just held on to her coat tails, and loved every second of it.

I can't imagine life without her, and I still can't believe she's gone. I know I was the luckiest man in the world to have loved and been loved by her. She gave us our beautiful daughter, who has been my strength through all of these dark days.

Some people leave behind great achievements to wonder at, and Bernie did just that; but I believe Bernie's greatest achievement is that no one has a bad word about her, and anytime any of us remember Bernie, I know we'll be smiling and remembering her beautiful smile and her unstoppable zest for life. We are all richer for having known her.

She lit up every room she ever walked into, and she

lit up my life forever. I'll love you for eternity Bernie, my beautiful girl.

It seems fitting to me that the last word should be from Bernie, and with that in mind, here is the message Bernie wrote to be read at her funeral. Once again it shows her love of life and an unbelievable absence of self-pity.

Hello everyone and thank you so much for coming. Don't be crying too much for me. Obviously I'd like a bit – I think I'm worth a little crying – but not too much.

No one has had a better life than me really - 50 years of singing some of the best ever shows including *Chicago*, *Blood Brothers*, *Sound of Music*, *My Fair Lady* and *City of Angels*. What an amazing time I have had.

By the time I was 19 I had been all over the world, sang with Stevie Wonder, toured with Frank Sinatra. . . I mean do not mourn my passing, CELEBRATE my wonderful life.

I have the most wonderful family who have supported me always, giving me great advice and constant love. As for my husband and daughter - how did I get so lucky?

Steve has been my constant rock, misunderstood terribly at times but if only you all knew what he has done for me and how he has set up Erin's life so she won't ever have to worry again, how he has cared for me and basically given up so much for me.

Every 17th October I want you to have a party, or at least a good old drink for my birthday. Make it vodka.

Acknowledgements

....

It's time to say thank you. This is going to read like another book!

Firstly, I want to mention my great friend Drew, who has stood by me from the very beginning. We wrote audition pieces together, choosing what songs to sing and what to wear. He was my rock. Thank you so very much, Drew.

A big thank you to Fenella Bates and all at my publishers Hodder & Stoughton. You have made it such a joy!

Big thanks and loads of love to Amanda Beckman – a truly lovely lady and a great agent, who has stood by me through everything. Thank you so much, Amanda. Thanks to Danielle – you are going to be a fab agent! A huge thank you to my wonderful manager and agent Neil Howarth. You have stood by me and totally supported me above and beyond the call of duty, Neil. We have had our ups and downs, but I always trusted your judgment. Thank you from the bottom of my heart! I love you.

Next, my wonderful fan club. Thank you all so much for your constant support and love, and for all your cards and letters. You really are a special bunch of people!

Now my family . . . what can I say? You have all supported me throughout my life, every step of the way with love and good advice. I could not have got through this life without you all. You have each played a major role and I love you all so very, very much.

Thank you to my wonderful parents – I think I have explained how I feel in the book!

To the amazing Claire Higney, who helped me put my story into words, a truly special woman and so very talented – I've had such fun with you over our lunches and teas. You make it all so easy. Thank you so very much.

A big thank you to Robert Kelly and Chris Jordan, two producers who have stood by me, allowing me to get better without having to worry. Thank you both so very much!

And now David Ian, a true friend who allowed me to take time off with a stupid cough and never made me feel bad about being off work. I really can't think of anything to say that would be enough. You have been truly wonderful. Thank you from the bottom of my heart, David.

I would also like to say a massive thank you to all at the Royal Surrey Hospital for the way they have looked after me. A special thank you to my oncologist Dr Stephen Houston, who has been fabulous, and my surgeon Mr Mark Kissin, who did a truly amazing job

Acknowledgements

(I have never seen such an amazing mastectomy!). Thanks to you both.

Another big thank you to my breast care nurses, especially to Olga, who went above and beyond. You always replied to my calls, never neglected me and did everything you could to help me. Thank you so very much, Olga, you are wonderful!

And thank God for the NHS. We truly are so very lucky in this country.

Finally, thank you to my husband and wonderful daughter. Steve, I can't believe how lucky I've been to have met you and for you to have fallen in love with me. No one could have looked after me better or made me feel so protected, loved and cherished. Thank you for 18 wonderful years of marriage, filled with fun, laughter and happiness.

Now, what do you say about a nearly 14-year-old-girl who is mature, wise and understanding beyond her years, and who has never given us a moment's trouble in her life? God, I have been so blessed. Thank you Erin, you are truly inspirational and have kept me going! I love you so, so much my darling daughter!

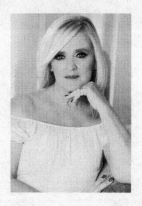

Bernie was a huge supporter of Breakthrough Breast Cancer, working with *Daybreak* to help raise awareness of Breakthrough's TLC (Touch Look Check) campaign. It's no exaggeration to say that her commitment to this cause, and the exposure she gave it, has helped to save lives. In honour of the amazing work Bernie did Breakthrough have decided to set up a fund in her name. If you would like to donate please visit www.breakthrough.org.uk/bernienolan.

An invitation from the publisher

Join us at www.hodder.co.uk, or follow us
on Twitter @hodderbooks to be a part of
our community of people who love the very
best in books and reading.

Whether you want to discover more about a book
or an author, watch trailers and interviews, have the
chance to win early limited editions, or simply browse
our expert readers' selection of the very best books,
we think you'll find what you're looking for.

And if you don't, that's the place to tell us what's missing.

We love what we do, and we'd love you to be a part of it.

www.hodder.co.uk

 @hodderbooks

HodderBooks

HodderBooks